Racial Stereotyping and Child Development

Contributions to Human Development

Vol. 25

Series Editor

Larry Nucci   Berkeley, Calif.

Racial Stereotyping and Child Development

Volume Editor

Diana T. Slaughter-Defoe Philadelphia, Pa.

2 figures and 4 tables, 2012

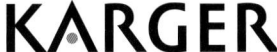

Basel · Freiburg · Paris · London · New York · New Delhi · Bangkok · Beijing · Tokyo · Kuala Lumpur · Singapore · Sydney

Diana T. Slaughter-Defoe
Graduate School of Education
The University of Pennsylvania
3700 Walnut Street
Philadelphia, PA 19104-6216, USA

Library of Congress Cataloging-in-Publication Data

Racial stereotyping and child development / editor, Diana T. Slaughter-Defoe.
     p. cm. -- (Contributions to human development ; v. 25)
  Includes bibliographical references and index.
  ISBN 978-3-8055-9982-5 (soft cover : alk. paper) -- ISBN 978-3-8055-9983-2
(electronic version)
   1. Child development. 2. Race awareness in children. 3. Ethnopsychology.
4. Identity (Psychology) and mass media. I. Slaughter-Defoe, Diana T.
  HQ767.9.R33 2012
  155.4--dc23
                                                   2012004301

Bibliographic Indices. This publication is listed in bibliographic services, including Current Contents®.

© Copyright 2012 by S. Karger AG, P.O. Box, CH–4009 Basel (Switzerland)
www.karger.com
Printed in Germany on acid-free and non-aging paper (ISO 9706) by Kraft Druck GmbH, Ettlingen
ISSN 0301–4193
e-ISSN 1664–2570
ISBN 978–3–8055–9982–5
e-ISBN 978–3–8055–9983–2

Contents

Introduction

Diana T. Slaughter-Defoe

University of Pennsylvania, Constance E. Clayton Professor Emerita in Urban Education, Graduate School of Education, University of Pennsylvania, Philadelphia, Pa., USA

Abstract

We know human biological diversity is occasioned by culture and ethnicity, not by race. There is as much or more variability within identified racial groups as there is between the 'racial' groups initially identified as humans entered the 20th century over 100 years ago. However, we also know that race, racial stratification, and racism continue today as enduring macro-societal variables in the lives of children, their families, and peers. Emphasizing the personal-social construction of race, scholars today prefer to study how children become racialized, inclusive of the contributions of political processes to the accompanying psychological development. Thus, racialization is construed as a situated process. Some scholars use the term 'colorism' to refer to various social practices used to racially stratify people informally. By definition, such stratification dictates individual cultural capital and resource allocation. This volume is partly designed to present and interrogate the research that some members of the Interdisciplinary Program in Human Development (ISHD) have conducted at the University of Pennsylvania, but more importantly, and by example, to stimulate theory and research on the topic of race and colorism by bringing together previously dispersed literature in a reader-friendly volume that highlights studies with promising concepts and methods.

Significance of the Concept of 'Race' to Developmental Inquiry

In the 21st century, scientists now know and acknowledge that the concept of race has no biogenetic basis [Cohen, 1998; Fisher, Jackson & Villarruel, 1998; Paabo, 2001; Segall, 1999]. Human biological diversity is occasioned by culture and ethnicity, not by race. There is as much or more variability within identified racial groups as there is between the 'racial' groups initially identified as humans entered the 20th century over 100 years ago. Further, this variability reaches deep into the previously thought homogeneous racial groups.

However, despite wishful thinking [e.g., Wilson, 1978], we know that race, racial stratification, and racism continue today as enduring macro-societal variables in the lives of children, their families, and peers. The legacy is particularly strong in cultures and nations (e.g., United States of America, South Africa) that have historically used race as an important, long-term principle of cultural and social organization [Franklin, 1968; Franklin, 1976; Franklin & Higginbotham, 2011; Gossett, 1970]. In such environments, children learn from caregivers and significant others how to cope with hostile racial environments [Chestang,

1972], while continuing to develop fully and to experience living normal and rich lives. The challenges of this paradox are now briefly discussed.

Historically, both the US and South Africa have experienced organized resistance to racism [American Psychological Association, 2004; Arsenault, 2006; Howard, 1970; King, 1969; Levander, 2006; Smiley, 2006], specifically, to the use of race as a major legal organizing societal principle (apartheid). Today, therefore, legal evidence of racial discrimination has been minimized, and even largely eliminated [Franklin, 1976]. However, the residue of earlier racial stratification endures [Bonilla-Silva & Lewis; Doane & Bonilla-Silva, 2003; Loury, 2002] and therefore, racial socialization is considered integral to the lives of all children in these cultures [Boykin & Toms, 1985; Clark & Klein, 2004; Hughes, Rodriguez, Smith, Johnson, Stevenson & Spicer, 2006; McAdoo, 2007; Ritterhouse, 2006; Slaughter & Johnson, 1988; Woodson, 1933].

Skin color/tone, or the presence of melanin, has been the most consistently used indicator of racial status in the US (for example, hair texture, linguistic surface features, evidence of prior racial blood lines have also been used) [Clark & Clark, 1939, 1940, 1947; Clark & Klein, 2004; Hunter, 2005; Porter, 1971]. Preschool-aged children first learn to reliably distinguish Black from White skin (racial awareness), and later to project or display certain attitudes toward the identified skin color or other race-related phenotypes. The racial attitudes are thought learned initially from family members [Goodman, 1952].

Colorism and Racial Stratification in the 21st Century

According to a very diverse body of scholars who study the impact of racial/color stratification for educational and occupational concerns, both in the US and abroad, skin color matters in this 21st century [Appiah & Gutmann, 1996; Bonilla-Silva & Lewis, 1999; Bonilla-Silva, 2001; Conchas, 2006; Cross, 1991; Dee, 2001; Dixson & Rousseau, 2006; Doane & Bonilla-Silva, 2003; Herring, Keith & Horton, 2004; Hilliard III, 2001; Hunter, 2005; Lee & Slaughter-Defoe, 2004; McLoyd, 2006; Nagda, Tropp & Paluck, 2006; Ogbu, 2003; Pollock, 2004; Spencer, 2006a, b; Watkins, 2001]. Issues raised by children's skin color and race and addressed by members of the Black Caucus of the Society for Research in Child Development (SRCD), continue to be addressed by the profession today [Slaughter-Defoe, Garrett & Harrison, 2006]. Indeed, a special issue devoted to race, ethnicity and culture in child development was published in a 2006 volume of *Child Development*, the premier journal in this field [Quintana, Aboud, Chao, Contreras-Grau, Cross & Hudley, 2006]. Also, as Tatum observed [1992, 1997], it continues to be difficult to talk about race or racism in schools and classrooms, and strong evidence of racial in-group preferential attitudes and behavior, particularly in the middle school years and beyond, endure [Nagda, Tropp & Paluck, 2006], as do parental and extended African-American family members' attempts to buffer their children from racism [McHale, Crouter, Kim, Burton, Davis & Dotterer, 2006]. Recent research suggests that all of this is made more complex by the predilections of children and youth to choose their own multiracial paths [Hitlin, Brown & Elder, 2006], and by the situated quality of racial designations and relations.

Emphasis on Black and White skin color as a symbol of racial identity in the 20th century has led to some contemporary confusion about African-American designation and identity in this 21st century. Not all persons who are in possession of darker skin and considered Black are Black American natives whose ancestors experienced racial injustice in America that extends back to the time prior to President Abraham Lincoln's Emancipation Proclamation. Further, biracial persons may or may not be able to claim this distinction. For example, President

Barack Obama [1995] cannot make this claim, but former US Congressman Harold Ford, Jr. of Memphis, who is light-skinned enough to appear biracial, can. Increased immigration to the US of darker-skinned peoples is likely to further confound distinctions between the children of more recent Black or darker-skinned immigrants, and those who can claim to be the children of Black or darker-skinned natives [Massey, Mooney, Charles & Torres, 2007]. Obviously, intergenerational transmission of ideas and attitudes regarding race and racism differ for these two broad cultural groups.

Colorism, focusing as it does on darker-skinned, non-White people of color, is thought by some to be a 'disease' created by global racism. In this 'affliction' usually the lighter, closer to white, the skin's color, the better, more highly valued, the wearer of the skin. Scholars like Bonilla-Silva believe that the waning of racial boundaries generated by apartheid policies is leading to heightened discrimination based on skin color. Therefore, not race, but its most enduring proxy, skin color within race, continues to pose the challenges originally described many years ago by Warner, Junker and Adams [1941].

Unlike Warner and colleagues, however, colorism theorists believe the phenomenon is an outgrowth of racism. Emphasizing the personal-social construction of race, these scholars prefer to study how children become racialized, and the contributions of political processes to the accompanying psychological development. Thus, racialization is construed as a situated process – the developing child is perceived as light or dark-skinned according to the immediate cultural or political environment in which s/he participates – a very light-skinned biracial child, for example, may simultaneously be the favored child in a family home environment, but a truly undervalued Black child in a desegregated suburban classroom.

To summarize, the concept 'colorism' references the various social practices used to filter and allocate people into different racial locations in the racial order, that is, social practices used to racially stratify people informally. By definition, such stratification dictates cultural capital and resource allocation.

Revisiting 'Race' in Current Developmental Research

In 2009, Professors Deborah Johnson, Margaret Beale Spencer, and I published a brief overview of existing knowledge about race and children's development in an encyclopedic compendium entitled *The Child,* edited by Richard Shweder and colleagues [Slaughter-Defoe, Johnson & Spencer, 2009]. Our entry was reinforced by an extensive bibliographic search and review that could not be published in that venue. Our search also revealed that the literature on this topic was quite dispersed, and therefore, that possibly both theory and empirical research in this area could be advanced by being brought together in a reader-friendly volume that highlights studies with promising concepts and methods. The new empirical studies presented in this volume take cognizance of the earliest research in race and child development, but advance its contemporary implications, given our current understanding of both development and social cognition.

The first report presented by Ms. Erin Bogan focuses on review of the developmental trajectories of racial stereotypes of Black and White children, examining the recent empirical research from the perspective of theorizing associated with experimental studies of stereotyped-threat [Steele & Aronson, 1995; Steele, 1997, 2004]. The second study, conducted by Dr. Valerie Adams, addresses the theoretical and empirical role of media images in influencing the race-related images Black children come to have of themselves. The third study, conducted by Dr. Traci English-Clarke, draws upon the PVEST theoretical model [Spencer, 2006a, b] in considering the significance of racial messages and stories for how children think of themselves as academically competent in mathematics, a field identified by activist educator Robert Moses [2001] as a gatekeeper to higher education. All studies by the primary authors were conducted at the University of Pennsylvania immediately prior to 2010, with the support and mentoring of secondary authors and collaborators.

The primary authors were influenced by the philosophy, methods, and practical orientation of the Interdisciplinary Studies in Human Development Program (ISHD) where this editor was a standing faculty member for 13.5 years through June 2011. The program emphasizes phenomenological development in context, inclusive of macro-societal and policy-relevant contexts, as well as the more traditional microsystemic and evaluative contexts. The interdisciplinary nature of the studies in chapters I–III occasioned the editor's intent of obtaining commentary to each of them from primarily senior and established scholars across different academic disciplines and fields, including subfields within the disciplines.

The article by Professor Nsamenang, an established scholar in the subfield of cultural psychology, demonstrates how far-reaching conceptions of race-related behavior can be even for the positive development of Black African children, who enjoy majority status in their own countries and continent. Instead of commentaries by established and publically recognized scholars in the broad fields of race and social psychological development as in the other chapters, commentaries for this informative concluding chapter are provided by two current doctoral students in ISHD.

Finally, the editor's Epilogue, or concluding, chapter points to ideas not fully developed by authors, and also highlights shared thematic content between sections.

Du Bois [1903] predicted race would be the problem of the 20th century, but research and commentary in this volume indicate that race and color endure as problems of the 21st century. For persons interested in race and children's development, this compendium of efforts to address the cultural/racial contexts of 21st century children and youth are both troubling and promising to the field of human development.

References

American Psychological Association WCAR Delegation (2004). *The United Nations World Conference against Racism, Racial Discrimination, Xenophobia and Related Intolerance* (WCAR), August 28–September 8, 2001. Durban, South Africa. Washington: American Psychological Association.

Appiah, A., & Gutmann, A. (1996). *Color conscious: The political morality of race*. Princeton: Princeton University Press.

Arsenault, R. (2006). *Freedom riders: 1961 and the struggle for racial justice*. Oxford: Oxford University Press.

Bonilla-Silva, E., & Lewis, A. (1999). The new racism: Toward an analysis of the US Social structure, 1960s–1990s. In P. Wong (Ed.), *Race, ethnicity, and nationality in the United States: Toward the twenty-first century* (Chapter 5). Boulder: Westview Publishers.

Bonilla-Silva, E. (2001). *White supremacy and racism in the post-civil rights era*. Boulder: Lynne Rienner Publishers.

Boykin, A.W., & Toms, F.D. (1985). Black child socialization: A conceptual framework. In H.P. McAdoo & J.L. McAdoo (Eds.), *Black children: Social, educational, and parental environments* (pp. 33–51). Thousand Oaks: Sage Publications, Inc.

Chestang, L. (1972). *Character development in a hostile environment*. Chicago: University of Chicago School of Social Service Administration.

Clark, K.B., & Clark, M.K. (1939). The development of consciousness of self and the emergence of racial identification in Negro preschool children. *Journal of Social Psychology, 10,* 591–599.

Clark, K.B., & Clark, M.K. (1940). Skin color as a factor in racial identification of Negro preschool children. *Journal of Social Psychology, 11,* 159–169.

Clark, K.B., & Clark, M.K. (1947). Racial identification and preference in Negro children. In T. Newcomb & E. Hartley (Eds.), *Readings in social psychology* (pp. 602–611). New York, NY: Holt.

Clark, K.B., & Klein, W. (2004). *Toward humanity and justice: The writings of Kenneth B. Clark, scholar of the 1954 Brown v. Board of Education decision*. Westport: Praeger.

Cohen, M.N. (1998). Culture, not race, explains human diversity. [Electronic version]. *Chronicle of Higher Education*, April 17, B4-B5. Retrieved 02/11/2007, from http://allrelated.syr.edu/resources.html database.

Conchas, G.Q. (2006). *The color of success: Race and high-achieving urban youth.* New York: Teachers College Press.

Cross, W.E.J. (1991). *Shades of black: Diversity in African-American identity.* Philadelphia: Temple University Press.

Dee, T. (2001). *Teachers, race and student achievement in a randomized experiment.* (NBER Working Paper No. W8432). Cambridge: National Bureau of Economic Research, Inc. Retrieved February 13, 2007, from http://www.nber.org/papers/W8432.

Dixson, A.D., & Rousseau, C.K. (2006). *Critical race theory in education: All God's children got a song.* New York: Routledge.

Doane, A.W., & Bonilla-Silva, E. (2003). *White out: The continuing significance of racism.* New York: Routledge.

Du Bois, W.E.B. (1903). *The souls of Black folk: Essays and sketches* (2nd ed.). Chicago: A.C. McClurg & co.

Fisher, C.B., Jackson, J.F., & Villarruel, F.A. (1998). The study of African American and Latin American children and youth. In W. Damon, et al. (Ed.), *Handbook of child psychology* (5th ed., pp. 1145–1208). New York: John Wiley & Sons.

Franklin, J.H. (1968). *Color and race.* Boston: Houghton Mifflin.

Franklin, J.H. (1976). *Racial equality in America.* Chicago: University of Chicago.

Franklin, J.H., & Higginbotham, E. (2011). *From slavery to freedom: A history of African Americans* (9th ed.). New York: McGraw-Hill.

Goodman, M.E. (1952). *Race awareness in young children.* Cambridge: Addison-Wesley Publishing Co.

Gossett, T.F. (1970). *Race: The history of an idea in America.* New York: Schocken Books.

Herring, C., Keith, V., & Horton, H.D. (2004). *Skin deep: How race and complexion matter in the 'color-blind' era.* Urbana: University of Illinois Press, Institute for Research on Race and Public Policy, University of Illinois at Chicago.

Hilliard III, A.G. (2001). 'Race', identity, hegemony, and education: What do we need to know now? In J. Watkins, J. Lewis & V. Chou (Eds.), *Race and education: The roles of history and society in educating African American students* (pp. 7–33). Boston: Allyn and Bacon.

Hitlin, S., Brown, J.S., & Elder, G.H.J. (2006). Racial self-categorization in adolescence: Multiracial development and social pathways. *Child Development, 77,* 1298–1308.

Howard, J.H. (1970). How to end colonial domination of Black America. *Negro Digest, 1,* 4.

Hughes, D., Rodriguez, J., Smith, E.P., Johnson, D.J., Stevenson, H.C., & Spicer, P. (2006). Parents' ethnic-racial socialization practices: A review of research and directions for future study. *Developmental Psychology, 42,* 747–770.

Hunter, M.L. (2005). *Race, gender, and the politics of skin tone.* New York: Routledge.

King, M.L. (1969). The role of the behavioral scientist in the civil rights movement. In N. Glenn & C. Bonjean (Eds.), *Blacks in the United States* (1st ed., pp. 3–12). San Francisco: Chandler.

Lee, C., & Slaughter-Defoe, D.T. (2004). Historical and sociocultural influences in African American education. In J.A. Banks & C.A.M. Banks (Eds.), *Handbook of research on multicultural education* (2nd ed., pp. 462–490). New York: Macmillan Publishing Co.

Levander, C.F. (2006). Cradle of liberty: Race, the child, and national belonging from Thomas Jefferson to W.E.B. Du Bois. Durham: Duke University Press.

Loury, G. (2002). *The anatomy of racial inequality.* Cambridge: Harvard University.

Massey, D., Mooney, M., Charles, C., & Torres, K. (2007). Black immigrants and black natives attending selective colleges and universities in the United States. *American Journal of Education, 113,* 243–271.

McAdoo, H.P. (2007). *Black families* (4th ed.). Thousand Oaks: Sage Publications.

McHale, S.M., Crouter, A.C., Kim, J., Burton, L.M., Davis, K.D., & Dotterer, A.M., et al. (2006). Mothers' and fathers' racial socialization in African American families: Implications for youth. *Child Development, 77,* 1387–1402.

McLoyd, V.C. (2006). The legacy of child development's 1990 special issue on minority children: An editorial retrospective. *Child Development, 77,* 1142–1148.

Moses, R. (2001). Radical equations: Civil rights from Mississippi to the Algebra Project. Boston: Beacon Press.

Nagda, B.A., Tropp, L., & Paluck, E.L. (2006). Reducing prejudice and promoting social inclusion: Integrating research, theory, and practice on intergroup relations. *Journal of Social Sciences, 62,* 439–451.

Obama, B. (1995). *Dreams from my father: A story of race and inheritance.* New York: Random House.

Ogbu, J.U. (2003). Black American students in an affluent suburb: A study of academic disengagement. Mahwah, NJ: L. Erlbaum Associates.

Paabo, S. (2001). The human genome and our view of ourselves. [Electronic version]. *Science, 291,* 1219–1220. Retrieved 02/11/2007, from http://allrelated.syr.edu/resources.html database.

Pollock, M. (2004). *Colormute: Race talk dilemmas in an American school.* Princeton: Princeton University Press.

Porter, J.D.R. (1971). *Black child, White child; the development of racial attitudes.* Cambridge: Harvard University Press.

Quintana, S.M., Aboud, F.E., Chao, R.K., Contreras-Grau, J., Cross, W.E.J., & Hudley, C., et al. (2006). Race, ethnicity, and culture in child development: Contemporary research and future directions. *Child Development, 77,* 1129–1141.

Ritterhouse, J.L. (2006). *Growing up Jim Crow: How Black and White Southern children learned race.* Chapel Hill: University of North Carolina.

Segall, M.H. (1999). Why is there still racism if there is no such thing as 'race'? In W.J. Lonner, D.L. Dinnel, D.K. Forgays & S.A. Hayes (Eds.), *Merging past, present, and future in cross-cultural psychology.* Lisse: Swets & Zeitlinger.

Slaughter-Defoe, D.T., Johnson, D.J., & Spencer, M.B. (2009). Race and children's development. In R.A. Shweder, T.R. Bidell, A.C. Dailey, S.D. Dixon, P.J. Miller & J. Modell (Eds.), *The child: An encyclopedic companion* (pp. 801–806). Chicago: University of Chicago Press.

Slaughter, D.T., & Johnson, D.J. (Eds.) (1988). *Visible now: Blacks in private schools.* New York: Greenwood Press.

Slaughter-Defoe, D.T., Garrett, A.M., & Harrison-Hale, A.O. (Eds.) (2006). Our children too: A History of the first 25 years of the Black Caucus of the Society for Research in Child Development, 1973–1997. *Monographs of the Society for Research in Child Development, 71*, 1, Serial No. 283. Boston: Blackwell.

Smiley, T. (2006). *The covenant with Black America* (1st ed.). Chicago: Third World Press, The Smiley Group.

Spencer, M.B. (2006b). Phenomenology and ecological systems theory: Development of diverse groups. In W. Damon & R. Lerner (Eds.), *Handbook of child psychology* (6th ed.): *Vol 15, Theoretical models of human development.* (pp. 829–893). Hoboken: John Wiley & Sons.

Spencer, M.B., Harpalani, V., Cassidy, E., Jacobs, C.Y., Donde, S., & Goss, T.N., et al. (2006a). Understanding vulnerability and resilience from a normative developmental perspective: Implications for racially and ethnically diverse youth. In D. Cicchetti & D.J. Cohen (Eds.), *Developmental psychopathology, Vol. 1: Theory and method* (2nd ed., pp. 627–672). Hoboken: John Wiley & Sons.

Steele, C.M. (2004). A threat in the air: How stereotypes shape intellectual identity and performance. In J.A. Banks & C.A.M. Banks (Eds.), *Handbook of research on multicultural education* (2nd ed., pp. 682–699). San Francisco: Jossey-Bass.

Steele, C.M., & Aronson, J. (1995). Stereotype threat and the intellectual test performance of African Americans. *Journal of Personality and Social Psychology, 69,* 797–811.

Steele, C.M. (1997). *Race and the schooling of Black Americans.* Upper Saddle River, NJ: Prentice-Hall, Inc.

Tatum, B.D. (1992). Talking about race, learning about racism: The application of racial identity development theory in the classroom. *Harvard Educational Review, 62,* 1–24.

Tatum, B.D. (1997). *'Why are all the black kids sitting together in the cafeteria?'* New York: Basic Books.

Warner, W., Junker, B., & Adams, W. (1941). *Color and human nature.* Washington: American Council on Education.

Watkins, W.H., Lewis, J.H., & Chou, V. (Eds.) (2001). *Race and education: The roles of history and society in educating African American students.* Boston: Allyn and Bacon.

Wilson, W.J. (1978). *The declining significance of race: Blacks and changing American institutions.* Chicago: University of Chicago Press.

Woodson, C.G. (1933). *The mis-education of the Negro.* Washington: Associated Publishers.

Prof. Diana T. Slaughter-Defoe
Graduate School of Education
University of Pennsylvania
3700 Walnut Street
Philadelphia, PA 19104–6216 (USA)
Tel. +1 215 582 7036
E-Mail dianasd@gse.upenn.edu

Dr. Diana T. Slaughter-Defoe (PhD 1968, University of Chicago) received her doctorate from the Committee on Human Development in developmental and clinical psychology, and is presently the Constance E. Clayton Professor Emerita in the Graduate School of Education at the University of Pennsylvania. Her research interests have included culture, primary education, and home-school relations facilitating in-school academic achievement. Since retirement, she has also edited: *Black Educational Choice: Assessing the Private and Public Alternatives to K-12 Public Schools* [Praeger, 2011] with colleagues, and *Messages for Educational Leadership: The Constance E. Clayton Lectures, 1998–2007* [Peter Lang Publishers, 2012]. She is presently writing a memoir about her career that spanned 40-plus years in academia and higher education.

Paper

Slaughter-Defoe DT (ed): Racial Stereotyping and Child Development.
Contrib Hum Dev. Basel, Karger, 2012, vol 25, pp 1–19

Through the Eyes of a Child: the Development and Consequences of Racial Stereotypes in Black and White Children

Erin D. Bogan[a] · Diana T. Slaughter-Defoe[b]

[a]University of Michigan, Ann Arbor, Mich., and [b]University of Pennsylvania, Philadelphia, Pa., USA

Abstract

This chapter provides an integrated review of research conducted on the formation of racial stereotypes in Black and White children and adolescents. Specifically, the chapter outlines the developmental trajectory in which these children and adolescents formulate racial stereotypes and compares how racial stereotypes impact children and adolescents in these two racial groups psychologically and socially. It focuses on longitudinal and cross sectional studies that compare the development of children over time and point to variations in age and gender. The chapter seeks to answer three questions: Research Question # 1: *What is the developmental trajectory of racial stereotypes in Black and White children?* Research Question # 2: *How do Black and White Children differ in the development of personal stereotypes and stereotype consciousness?* Research Question # 3: *What are the consequences related to the development of stereotypes in Black and White children?* Results from studies reviewed reveal that Black children are disproportionately negatively impacted by the development of racial stereotypes, particularly because of their advanced awareness of broadly held stereotypes. Results showing the variation in impact give insight into factors contributing to the racial achievement gap, and implications for stereotype threat interventions.

Copyright © 2012 S. Karger AG, Basel

This chapter reviews literature on the development of stereotypes in Black and White children between 1980 and 2010. The first author chose to focus on studies after 1980 because early studies focused primarily on the development of personal stereotypes, particularly by implementing forced choice techniques used in the Clark and Clark doll studies to examine racial preference. Prior to 1980, few studies were developmental. Many simply focused on preference and prejudice as they correlated with measures of childhood self-esteem. The studies ignored the developmental changes in racial attitudes that occur through adolescence. In addition, few studies took into account cognitive factors related to stereotype development until the mid-1970s, when many researchers began to conceptualize stereotyping as a normative cognitive process allowing one to simplify and synthesize new information. For these reasons, only studies published after 1980 were considered. Studies published after 1980 have built upon prior research and considered both cognitive and social factors related to the development of stereotypes in children.

For decades, the concept of 'stereotype' has been debated by researchers in the fields of social

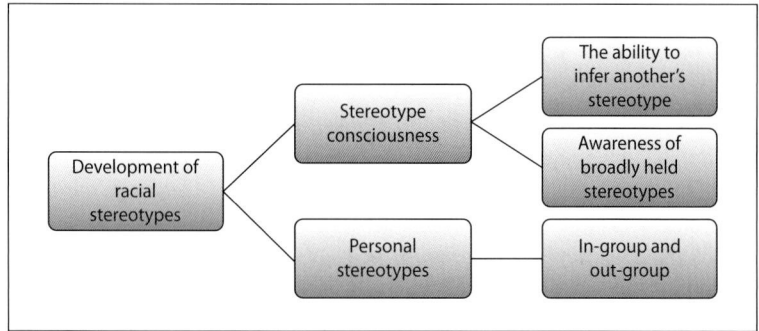

Fig. 1. Logic model.

and cognitive psychology. The concept of stereotyping is equally well known in both political and journalistic arenas. Generally, a stereotype can be defined as 'a set of beliefs about the personal attributes of a group of people' [Ashmore & Del Boca, 1981, p. 16]. Approaches in cognitive psychology have highlighted the important function stereotypes play, generally, in that they are 'categories that bring coherence and order to our social environment' and can help minimize the amount of information that we need to process [McGarty, Yzerbyt & Spears, 2002, p. 5].

While stereotypes generally aid us in our cognitive functioning, racial stereotypes can have a more deleterious impact, particularly on children. Results from studies of racial awareness and racial stereotypes suggest that the development of racial stereotypes in children may be more complicated in that Black and White children show different patterns of development. The patterns lead to different consequences, particularly in educational settings [McKown & Weinstein, 2003].

Different aspects of children's development of stereotypes have been studied and assessed from various perspectives. There are two facets of stereotype development that explain the development of racial stereotypes in Black and White children: personal stereotypes and stereotype consciousness. A personal stereotype is defined by McKown and Weinstein [2003] as 'children's own stereotypic beliefs' [p. 498] – stereotypes that

they endorse and believe. McKown and Weinstein [2003] explain that 'children who themselves believe that Whites are smarter than Blacks endorse a personal stereotype' [p. 489]. Children develop personal stereotypes about their in-group and various out-groups. Simultaneously, children are developing stereotype consciousness, or 'the awareness that others endorse stereotypes' [McKown & Weinstein, 2003, p. 489]. Two distinct features of stereotype consciousness have been identified by McKown and Weinstein [2003]: the first is the child's 'ability to infer another individual's stereotypes', and the second is the child's 'awareness of broadly held stereotypes' [McKown & Weinstein, 2003, p. 500].

In 1995, Claude Steele and Joshua Aronson, both experimental social psychologists, advanced theory and research suggesting that the salience of racial stereotypes, particularly in school settings, may negatively impact Black children psychologically, emotionally, and academically. However, few studies have linked the development of stereotypes to stereotype threat.

For this chapter, the first author examined the literature that pertains to both the development of personal stereotypes of in-groups and out-groups, and stereotype consciousness in these two groups – the two components of stereotype development (fig. 1).

According to McKown and Weinstein [2003], children simultaneously develop the ability to infer another individual's stereotype and awareness of broadly held stereotypes, as well as personal stereotypes about their in-group and out-group members.

Given the empirical data presented in this review three research questions guided the analyses:

(1) *What is the developmental trajectory of racial stereotypes in Black and in White children?*

(2) *How do Black and White children differ in the development of personal stereotypes and stereotype consciousness?*

(3) *What are the consequences related to the development of stereotypes in Black and White children?*

Background

Prior to presenting the method of this review, and the findings of the 14 identified empirical studies relative to these questions, a brief overview of critical pre-1980 research is presented in this Background section of the chapter.

In the late 1930s Clark and Clark [1939, 1940] conducted 'doll tests' in which the researchers showed individual Black children a Black doll and a White doll, following which they asked the children attitudinal questions about the dolls such as 'which doll is nicer', and 'which doll is prettier'. Afterwards, they asked each child being examined to identify the doll that looked most like herself (himself). Like their White peers, young Black children from segregated schools overwhelmingly showed a preference for the White dolls, even though the majority of children of both races accurately identified the doll that looked most like themselves.

For many years after the Clark and Clark studies purported to demonstrate linkages between racial attitudes and preferences and Black and White children's self-concepts and self-esteem, researchers focused on the methodological issues related to the early research. Research designs and measures were improved,

but assumptions remained largely unexamined until the 1970s when there was a significant amount of research produced that examined racial stereotypes in Black and White children [Spencer, 1982]. Early studies of adults such as those conducted and reported in Kardiner and Ovessey's [1951] *Mark of Oppression* suggested that Black children's awareness of race and racial preferences were linked to an inherent self-hate and low self-esteem. However, later studies that replicated the findings of the Clark and Clark doll test indicated that while Black children did develop Eurocentric racial attitudes, this dominant culture preference could have resulted from the children's heightened awareness of societal stereotypes, rather than originate as reflections of low self-esteem. Particularly when measures of self-concept and esteem were separately administered together with measures of racial attitudes and preferences [e.g., Crocker, 2000; Spencer, 1982], this newer possibility emerged. These findings and interpretations lead to new studies designed to examine the complexity of the development of children's racial stereotypes, and to identify factors that explain why Black and White children might develop stereotypes differently.

Method of Review

Types of Studies
Studies designed to show the development of racial stereotypes in children were either cross-sectional, longitudinal, or combined both approaches. A cross-sectional study is commonly used in developmental research to examine two or more samples within a population at a given period of time. A longitudinal study, also common in developmental research, looks at the same population or sample in at least two given points of time. Only cross-sectional or longitudinal studies published between 1980 and 2010 were reviewed for this chapter.

Search Strategies Used to Identify the Studies
A 'snowball' technique was used in that the first author initially identified one study by McKown and Weinstein [2003] that specifically examined the development of

stereotype consciousness and consequences related to this development as well as another by Aboud and Skerry [1984]. Aboud and Skerry reviewed studies pertaining to the development of ethnic attitudes. Several key studies cited in those two articles, as well as key terms, were identified for further examination.

The PsychInfo Database was also used to search key terms with restrictions to date (1980–2010), age (<12 years old), race (Black or White or both Black and White), and study type (cross-sectional or longitudinal). The following were key terms that yielded results for the 14 studies identified: racial stereotypes, racial attitudes, racial preference, ethnic attitudes, ethnic bias, racial bias, bias, prejudice, self-awareness, self-identification, ethnic identification, ethnic self-awareness, racial awareness, in-group attitudes, out-group attitudes, in-group racial attitudes, out-group racial attitudes, stereotype awareness, stereotype threat, and stereotype formation.

During the searches, studies were evaluated to ensure they met the criteria for preferred types of studies. Once the 14 studies were identified, an outline was created for each study to organize the content and identify the independent and dependent variables, as well as the measures and findings. A separate outline was created which organized the developmental sequences from the data presented in each study for later analysis. Data and details from each study were then analyzed from the perspective of the three research questions.

Of the studies obtained through the various searches, 14 were found that pertained to the development of racial stereotypes in Black and White children (table 1).

Of these 14 studies, 6 included samples of Black children, 5 included samples of White children and 3 included samples of both Black and White children. All studies included both male and female children. Some studies involved children of other racial/ethnic groups. However, this chapter addresses only findings related to Black and White children. The 14 studies provided empirical data on a total of 2,198 children.

Using the PsychInfo Database, the first author conducted a search for biracial children and stereotype development. This search yielded 724 references. However, most of these studies appeared to focus on racial identity and less on the actual development of stereotypes, so they were excluded from present analyses.

Types of Participants
Participants in the studies reviewed were Black and White children. Some studies included children of other ethnicities; however, results pertaining to these children were not included in the analysis. Children ranged between 3 and 12 years of age; they attended preschool through 6th grade.

Types of Outcome Measures
Studies focused primarily on in-group and out-group preference, bias, racial attitudes, and prejudice in Black and White children, and the ability to infer another individual's stereotypes and the awareness of broadly held stereotypes. Studies also measured social affect towards various racial cues and stimuli. Likewise, level of cognitive development was measured in some studies in order to draw comparisons between changes in racial attitudes and various cognitive abilities, and test performances. Self-concept was also measured in studies, as well as factors known to be related to the effects of stereotype threat, such as anxiety.

Results and Discussion

Research Question # 1: What Is the Developmental Trajectory of Racial Stereotypes in Black and White Children?
Black Children's Development of Personal Stereotypes
Racial preference has been found in preschool aged Black children as young as 3 years old [Spencer, 1982]. According to Semaj [1980], the greatest variability in Black children's racial evaluations occurs during early preschool ages. Black children under ages 4–5 years old attribute positive evaluations to both Black and White racial stimuli with no consistent racial preference. However, according to the research literature, Black children generally begin to show an out-group preference for Whites during the preschool years [Semaj, 1980; Spencer, 1982, 1984]. Children between ages 4–5 years show a Eurocentric orientation in preference attitudes and color concepts demonstrated through their 'evaluative statements about Black or White persons (i.e. children); preference statements about the child's choice of friends, classmates, playmates, studymates' [Spencer, 1982, p. 78].

Spencer [1984] found that 73% of Black children in her preschool aged sample showed race dissonance, that is, White-biased or Eurocentric preferences [Spencer, 1984]. This development was found to be particularly prominent,

Table 1. Studies pertaining to the development of racial stereotypes in Black and White children

Study	Cross-sectional (CS) or longitudinal (L)	Sample size, n	Race Black (B) White (W) other (O)	Age range	Gender
Abound, 1980	CS	99	B = 32 W = 67	5.17–7.10	Black: 15 = M, 15=F White: 36 = M, 31=F
Averhart & Bigler, 1997	CS	56	B = 56	5.9–7.4	not available
Branch & Newcombe, 1986	L and CS	51	B = 51	4–7	M = 21, F = 30
Bigler & Liben, 1993	CS	75	W = 75	4–9	not available
Clark, Hocevar, & Dembo, 1980	L and CS	72	W = 72	2.5–10.5	not available
Davey & Mullin, 1980	CS	512	B = 128 W = 256 O = 128	7–10	not available
Doyle & Abound, 1995	L and CS	96	W = 96	5.9–8.9	time 1: M = 44, F = 52 time 2: M = 20, F = 27
Doyle, Beaudet, & Abound, 1988	CS	232	W = 232	5–11	M = 114, F = 118
McKown & Weinstein, 2003 (Study 1)	CS	202	B, W and O	6–10	not available
McKown & Weinstein, 2003 (Study 2)	CS	202	B, W and O	6–10	not available
Semaj, 1980	CS	80	B = 80	4–11	M = 35, F = 45
Spencer, 1982	CS	384	B = 384	3–9	not available
Spencer, 1984	CS	130	B = 130	4–6	not available
Williams & Davidson, 2009	CS	80	B = 76	6–11.2	M = 37, F = 39
Zinser, Rich & Bailey, 1981	CS	133	W = 133	5.58–10.59	M = 69, F = 64

with relatively positive evaluations of Whites, in younger preschool aged children. About 20% of the preschool children were nonbiased or neutral in their racial preferences. Overall, the majority of young Black children preferred White children to their own racial group.

Spencer [1984, p. 440] states that '. . .eighty% of the sample [of 130 preschool aged Black children] obtained positive self-concept scores, while demonstrating pro-White biased cultural values on a racial attitude and preference measure'. For boys ages 4 to 4.7, however, an increase in White bias or preferences was significantly related to an increase in self-concept. Contrary to Spencer's [1982] findings that suggested Black preschoolers' self-concept remains generally positive despite a White preference; however, Spencer [1984] found that, in 4- to 4.7-year-old girls and 4.8- to 5-year-old boys, as pro-White racial attitudes (White bias) increased, level of self-concept decreased. Generally, however, findings indicated that Black preschool children show a Eurocentric racial preference, but not low self-esteem. Spencer [1984] also found that preschool aged children young as 4 years old have racial attitudes that favored Whites. This White bias was found to be stronger in Black children who were more racially aware. For younger children and girls, White preference was directly predicted by race awareness.

In addition, early developmental patterns of racial attitudes and preference in Black preschool children are related to varying socioeconomic income statuses. Middle-income children were found to have a Eurocentric orientation on all dimensions measuring color concepts, racial attitudes, and racial preference at age 3 [Spencer, 1982]. Low-income children, however, obtained scores on these measures at age 3 that were neutral. After age 3, both low-income and middle-income children '. . .demonstrated a clear Eurocentric orientation for color concepts' [Spencer, 1982, p. 79]. Likewise, children from one-parent households showed a significantly greater White preference than children from two parent households [Branch & Newcombe, 1986].

Averhart and Bigler's [1997] study support the findings of White bias in Black children. Five-year-old Black children showed a Eurocentric preference, selecting a higher number of light-skinned dolls as well as lighter-complexioned individuals for teachers and playmates. Likewise, young Black children in this age group showed a better memory for stories that depicted dark-skinned individuals in a negative light and light-skinned individuals positively [Averhart & Bigler, 1997]. In addition, younger children saw light-skinned individuals as having higher occupational roles.

Only one study found contrasting patterns of development in young Black children. Aboud [1980] found that a majority of Black children had an in-group preference that did not change over time. Aboud [1980] did, however, find Black preschoolers who showed a White preference related to self-concept. Almost all of the children

in the study obtained self-concept scores that indicated a positive self-concept. Children's average self-concept scores were similar whether children were from the northern or southern regions of the United States. Fewer than 20% of the preschool children sampled had negative self-concepts. Of the 17 negative self-concept cases, 13 were also Eurocentric in orientation and represented 76% of all low self-concept cases. Only one child was found to have both Afrocentric racial attitudes and negative self-concept.

These White biases, however, were not found to be as significant in 7-year-olds, suggesting that White or Eurocentric preference in Black children begins to decrease by ages 5 and 6 [Averhart & Bigler, 1997; Spencer, 1984].

After age 5, children begin to develop an Afrocentric or pro-Black orientation that continues through age 9 [Semaj, 1980; Spencer, 1982]. In support of Spencer's [1982, 1984] findings that middle age periods are characterized by a decrease in White preference, Branch and Newcombe [1986] found that young Black children's out-group preference, exhibited at ages 4 and 5, begins to decrease. Black 6- and 7-year-old girls from two-parent households showed more Black preference than 4- and 5-year-old girls from two-parent households, suggesting that between ages 5 and 6, children gradually begin to develop more of an in-group preference. Similarly, 6- to 7-year-old Black children identified more Black dolls as having positive traits in a doll selection tests measuring racial preference than did 4- and 5-year-olds. In addition, 6- to 7-year-olds attributed fewer negative traits to Black dolls than White dolls by comparison to 4- to 5-year-olds [Branch & Newcomb, 1986].

Semaj [1980] also found the evaluation of Black stimulus by 6- and 7-year-old Black children becomes more positive of Blacks and more neutral towards Whites. Like Semaj [1980], Williams and Davidson [2009] found that children in this age range were neutral in remembering stereotype-consistent and stereotype-inconsistent information, again showing White bias had decreased. Children were more neutral and held no bias in that they were more likely to remember positive stories or negative stories, regardless of the race of the protagonist [Williams & Davidson, 2009]. Seven-year-olds gave a greater number of nonstereotyped answers, attributing both positive and negative attributes to both Black and White individuals [Averhart & Bigler, 1997]. Between the ages of 6 and 9 years, Black children's response patterns indicative of in-group preferences become more polarized towards Blacks [Semaj, 1980]. Likewise, Black children between the ages 8–9 had exhibited higher PRAM scores indicating more positive Black evaluations than younger children [Semaj, 1980]. In summary, the findings indicate that pro-White preference in Black children decreases over time as in-group attitudes become more positive up to age 9 [Branch & Newcombe, 1986; Semaj, 1980; Spencer 1982, 1984].

However, other findings suggest that there is *no* decrease of pro-White preference in Black children during this period. Williams and Davidson's [2009] findings indicate that at age of 9, Black children remembered more stereotype-consistent stories, a memory pattern indicating children at this age hold a pro-White bias and continue to endorse negative stereotypes about Blacks. Whites were chosen more frequently to have positives traits than any other group. Negative traits in hypothetical characters were less likely to be attributed to Whites. Black groups were chosen most likely to have negative traits. The findings were consistent along lines of age and gender [Williams & Davidson, 2009]. Similar patterns of bias were found with regard to skin color in this sample of Black 7- to 9-year-olds.

Positive traits were ascribed to light-skinned Blacks, while negative traits were more frequently said to be reflective of darker-complexioned Blacks [Williams & Davidson, 2009]. Findings form Davey and Mullin [1980] support Williams and Davidson's findings in that, in a sample of

128 Black children, fewer than 50% made own-race choices and preferred their race. Only 7- to 10-year-old boys demonstrated decreased pro-White preferences over time [Davey & Mullin, 1980]. Unlike Semaj [1980] and Branch and Newcombe [1986] who found a decrease in strong White preference, Davidson and Williams [2009] found that between the ages of 7 and 9 in-group attitudes about Blacks were generally negative and did not change significantly over time.

There is some evidence that this pattern of Black children's increasing positive in-group attitudes and decreases in White out-group attitudes changes again around age 10 and 11. Racial attitudes in Black children in this age range become neutral after having increased and decreased [Semaj, 1980]. In a sample of 10- and 11-year-olds, Semaj [1980] found that Black children exhibited equivalent positive evaluations to both Black and White stimuli. Results also indicated that Black children's pro-White preference increases at ages 10 and 11 after having declined from ages 4 to 9 years [Semaj, 1980]. More studies are needed to determine a clear pattern of development in older Black children during both the early and later adolescent years.

White Children's Development of Personal Stereotypes
Young White children were found to have a pro-White preference [Clark, Hocevar & Dembo, 1980; Zinser, Rich & Bailey, 1981]. This White bias is found in White preschool children as early as 4 years old. At age 4, White children were found to make in-group skin color choices [Clark et al., 1980]. Zinser, Rich and Bailey [1981] also found that younger White children, preschoolers and first graders (and some third graders), had a significantly greater in-group preference than any other age group. Similarly, Doyle and Aboud found that 85% of White kindergarteners were biased against Blacks. Likewise, preschoolers and first graders showed a significant preference for Whites, as they were the least likely to share with

Black children in hypothetical testing situations [Zinser et al., 1981]. Children in this age group also remembered stereotype-consistent stories more than stories that ran counter to stereotypes, and responded to 18 of the 24 PRAM questions measuring racial bias in a stereotypic way [Bigler & Liben, 1993]. In summary, these findings point to an early White bias in preschool aged White children.

These early manifestations of racial preference have been found to increase in White children up to 7 or 8 years of age [Clark et al., 1980; Zinser et al., 1981]. Researchers have found that children 5 years old to between 7 and 7.25 years old show more White bias than White children 5 years old or younger [Clark et al., 1980; Doyle et al., 1988]. Similarly, Zinser et al. [1981] found that in-group preference in White children significantly increased from ages 5 to 8. Among White children, this pro-White/anti-Black preference or bias remained consistently high from ages 3 to 10 in testing conditions with White examiners [Zinser et al., 1981].

Racial attitudes and preferences become more neutral in older White children [Doyle & Aboud, 1995; Doyle et al., 1988]. Doyle and Aboud [1995] found that by age 9, there were no differences in the positive and negative evaluations White children gave to hypothetical Black and White characters. At this age, attitudes towards Whites did not significantly change. However, attitudes towards Blacks were found to become more positive. This counter-bias was documented to occur between the ages of 6 and 9, such that by 9 years old, White children were no longer considered 'prejudiced' according to the PRAM racial preference tests [Doyle & Aboud, 1995]. White children, ages 8 and 10, show little racial preference in most hypothetical social situations [Zinser et al., 1980]. Ten-year olds show even less White bias than 8-year-olds. Zinser et al. [1980] suggest this is evidence of a decrease in pro-White preference over time. Similarly, Doyle et al. [1988] found little pro-White racial preference among White children ages 10–12. Children were able to ascribe both positive and negative characteristics to both hypothetical Black and White characters [Doyle et al., 1988]. Doyle and Aboud [1995], however, suggest the changes in older White children's racial attitudes do not indicate that bias has decreased, but instead that the children have acquired additional attitudes that run counter to prejudice. An example of this idea is a child who loves to play basketball. The child loves to play basketball so much that they are not concerned with who they play, or the race of their partner, as long as they get to play. White children maintain a preference in the direction of Whites, but the preference is not as strong as the preferences of younger White children [Bigler & Liben, 1993; Zinser et al., 1981].

Black and White Children's Development of Stereotype Consciousness

The only study to date that has examined stereotype consciousness in children is the McKown and Weinstein [2003] study. McKown and Weinstein [2003, p. 505] suggest that 'children become better at inferring others' specific social beliefs after age 6'. Their findings were supported by this idea in that between the ages of 6 and 10, children's ability to infer an individual's stereotype (stereotypes that they perceive other to hold) increases dramatically. Children 'move from virtually no awareness of other's stereotypes to being able to infer an individual's stereotype, to awareness of broadly held stereotypes' [McKown & Weinstein, 2003, p. 511]. Greater age, but not stigma status predicted greater likelihood of children inferring an individual's stereotype. This means regardless of race or gender, the time of onset for children being able to infer other's stereotype is the same for all children – 6 years old. Specifically, by 6 years 18% of children could infer an individual's stereotypes; this ability increased to 39% by age 7, 64% by age 8, and 83% by age 9. By age 10, 93% of children could infer another's stereotype. Therefore, substantial numbers of children gain the ability to infer another individual's stereotype by age 6, and over time this ability is shared by greater numbers of children.

In their 2003 paper, McKown and Weinstein also reported that children develop an awareness of broadly held stereotypes as early as age 6. According to McKown and Weinstein [2003, p. 506], 'When a child has developed the ability to infer another individual's stereotype, indirect evidence of others' behavior becomes available to the child'. They go on to explain that '. . .with a broader range of available evidence about other's stereotypes, the likelihood that children will learn about broadly held stereotypes increases'. Overall findings indicated that 85% of children who were aware of broadly held stereotypes could infer an individual's stereotype.

Similar to the development of the ability to infer another individual's stereotype is the developing awareness of broadly held stereotypes. This awareness increases with age so that by age 10 most children, despite race or gender, have some awareness of broadly held stereotypes. Children from academically stigmatized ethnic groups (e.g., Blacks and Latinos), however, were found to be more aware of broadly held stereotypes at all ages than children from academically nonstigmatized ethnic groups (e.g., Whites and Asians). Specifically, at age 6, 15% of Black (and Latino) children were aware of broadly held stereotypes versus 7% of White (and Asian) children. Similarly, for Blacks and Latinos, versus Whites and Asians, these figures were: at age 7, 28 versus 14%; at age 8, 46 versus 27%; at age 9, 65 versus 44%; and at age 10, 80 versus 63%.

Research Question # 2a: How Do Black and White Children Differ in the Development of Personal Stereotypes?
Preschool Age
A majority of the empirical studies indicated that, during preschool years, most Black children have an out-group preference [Averhart & Bigler, 1997; Branch & Newcombe, 1986; Spencer, 1984, 1982]. White children in the preschool age range overwhelming showed an in-group preference [Aboud, 1980; Clark et al., 1980; Davey & Mullin, 1980; Doyle et al., 1988; Zinser et al., 1981]. While there was a clear out-group preference in the studies presented about Black children's racial attitudes, White children's early in-group preference was referred to as an orientation towards their own group [Zinser et al., 1981].

Specifically, with regard to hypothetical situations related to close social distance, most young White children preferred their in-group [Zinser et al., 1981]. None of the White children in the study, however, provided a large number of responses that indicated the rejection of the child not selected as a recipient of sharing or companionship, as much as an overemphasis of positive qualities and feelings towards the selected child. While White children overall did show a White preference, answers from children indicated that this was, nevertheless, an orientation towards Whites rather than a strong preference. Likewise, answers did not indicate negative feelings towards the Black child that was not chosen and negative evaluations decreased with age. Black children, on the other hand, showed early strong out-group preferences demonstrated by preference for White or lighter skin individuals, more positive rating of White individuals over Blacks, as well the selection of Whites over Blacks in hypothetical situations [Spencer, 1984, 1982; Averhart & Bigler, 1997; Branch & Newcombe, 1986; Williams & Davidson, 2009]. These preferences in Black children, however, were characterized by negative views of Black [Williams & Davidson, 2009]. Only one study found that preschool aged children (Black children) did not show a racial preference [Semaj, 1980]. Overall, Black children have a White, out-group preference, while White children have an ethnocentric in-group preference prior to beginning kindergarten.

Increases and Decreases in Preference

Studies show that racial attitudes and preference, in both Black and White children, change and become stronger, more neutral, or decrease during certain periods of their development. Generally, studies showed that White children's out-group and in-group preferences will decrease over time, as the child matures [Aboud, 1980; Bigler & Liben, 1993; Doyle et al. [1988]; Doyle & Aboud, 1995; Zinser et al., 1981].

Doyle and Aboud [1995] and Clark et al. [1980], for example, found that as children get older, by around age 9, they are no longer categorized as prejudiced by the Preschool Racial Attitudes Measure (PRAM). In addition, this decrease in prejudice and in-group bias is not solely an increase in favorable out-group attitudes. Rather, it is characterized by counter-bias, that is, 'positive evaluations of out-groups and negative evaluations of other groups' [Aboud & Doyle, 1995, p. 223]. Counter-bias was a common theme in many of the studies presented. White children in these studies were able to maintain their ethnocentric preference for their in-group while acquiring 'additional attitudes that run counter to prejudice' [Aboud & Doyle, 1995, p. 223]. This counter bias is demonstrated by White children's ability to ascribe some positive qualities to out-group members and some negative qualities to in-group members. In-group preference, however, did not change [Aboud, 1980].

According to Doyle and Aboud [1995], 'single response measures of prejudice, which typically decrease with age (e.g., the Preschool Racial Attitude Measure – PRAM II) have been criticized for yielding only one index that confounds acceptance of one group with rejection of the other' [p. 210]. Aboud and Doyle [1995, p. 210] go on to explain that 'because only one race can be selected for each positive and negative evaluation, it is unclear whether the observed decrease in prejudice with age reflects a decrease in ethnocentric bias or an increase in attitudes that run counter to bias'.

To avoid this confound, Doyle et al. [1988] used multiple response measures. Doyle et al. [1988] found that with age, a flexibility in thinking or counter-bias did develop, and is demonstrated by the positive out-group evaluations and by negative in-group evaluations presented by White first through sixth graders. Bigler and Liben [1993] replicated these findings with White children between the ages of 4 and 9 years old. Bigler and Liben [1993] also found a pattern of counter-bias that develops in White children with age. Negative evaluations were given to both in-group and out-group members showing an overall decrease in in-group and out-group preference, while feelings towards in-group remained higher than those towards out-group members. In summary, White children's preferences do decrease with age, but remain favorable towards Whites.

Studies with Black children, on the other hand, yield more inconsistent conclusions regarding increases and decreases in preferences overtime. Williams and Davidson [2009] found that Black children maintained a White preference and negative in-group attitudes over time. These findings were supported by Aboud [1980] who found that in- group attitudes remained relatively stable over time. Although Aboud [1980] found a slight decline in-group preference, this trend was not significant. White preference, however, was shown to increase over time in Black children [Aboud, 1980]. Averhart and Bigler [1997] found that Black children's in-group preferences and out-group preferences both decreased over time.

Aboud's [1980] findings, however, were consistent with Semaj's [1980, p. 77] finding that Black children, with age, 'still [believe] "Black" is good, but are now either forced to or are more willing to accept that "White" is also good'. Semaj found that in-group preference increased between 6 and 9 years old but eventually decreased, as children got older. Black children's out-group evaluations, after decreasing between the ages of 6 and 9, also eventually increased over time. Semaj [1980, p. 77] suggests, however, 'perhaps as a result of an increasing number of experiences with prejudice, the child begins to lose some of the naturally positive identification with Blackness achieved at an early age'. Similar to White children's development of counter bias, Black children's preference, though stronger for out-group than in-group members, also becomes less polarized towards a particular group in that children begin to see both positive and negative aspects in Black and White individuals. Semaj [1980, p. 77] describes the uneasiness and hesitation that Black children demonstrated while having to choose between Black and White results from their 'increased ability to consider more than one aspect of a situation simultaneously'.

Preferences fluctuated more over time in Back children, but remained higher towards Whites than their own group whether or not they increased or decreased.

Cognitive Development
Clark et al. [1980] found that pro-White bias, or preference, was significantly lower in White children with higher levels of cognitive development when the examiner was Black. Children in the study were examined individually on four developmental measures and one skin color attitude measure, the Preschool Racial Attitude Measure (PRAM). The developmental measures included Piaget's clay and water task, the origin of night interview, the picture task and the skin color probe. Findings indicated stage-related abilities such as the developmental of physical conservation, comprehension of physical causality, and conservation of social identity were critical factors in children's understanding of ethnic differences. Children who scored higher on tests measuring these cognitive developments had a more accurate understanding of skin color and ethnic differences. Therefore, as they mature, children are beginning to understand that ethnicity is constant and not based on superficial features.

Clark et al. [1980] suggest, however, that these cognitive developments that allow for a better understanding of race may account for the apparent decrease in White- preference in older White children. Specifically, Clark et al. [1980] found that cognitive-developmental decreases in White preference were associated with a Black examiner, but not a White examiner. This suggests that as White children get older, they develop cognitively and begin to understand the implications of racial categories and, therefore, learn how to give socially desirable answers. Clark et al. [1980, p. 338] explains that the decrease in White children's pro-White preference may be a result of children 'responding the way they feel they are expected to', instead of an actual change in feelings towards other racial groups. According to Clark et al. [1980, p. 338], this perspective is not only supported by other studies, but by the fact that Black examiners are associated with 'decreases in pro-White bias with older children but not with younger White children'. In addition, 'age decreases are not found on less obtrusive measures of prejudice in which socially desirable responses are less obvious'. Finally, 'the decrease in pro-White bias associated with Black examiners is predominantly in children who are at higher levels of cognitive development'.

Similarly, Doyle and Aboud [1995] found that by third grade, children have developed enough cognitively to be able to ascribe both positive evaluations to out-group members and negative evaluations of their in-group. These counter-bias developments may 'allow older children to inhibit automatic biased evaluations during cross-race judgments and interactions' [p. 224].

However, although Doyle and Aboud [1995, p. 224] acknowledge that 'social desirability concerns are most likely to reduce negative evaluations of Black people', they found that no correlation between prejudice scores and scores on the Crandall Children's Social Desirability Scale concluding that it was 'unlikely that developmental changes in socially desirable responding account for the developmental change observed in prejudice' or preference in White children [Doyle &

Aboud, 1995, p. 224]. Doyle and Aboud [1995] did suggest that the development of social-cognitive skills were related to the reduction of prejudice in White children over time in that a relationship was found between increases in counter-bias and reconciliation. Children who understood that racial preferences could both be correct had greater increases in attitudes that ran counter to their White preference [Doyle & Aboud, 1995]. Researchers state that 'findings support Piaget's view that only when perspective taking includes the reconciliation of different perspectives is it accompanied by an understanding that there may be some positive qualities in other groups worth liking' [Doyle & Aboud, 1995, p. 225]. In support of this idea, results indicated that older children were more likely to change their racial preference ratings to make them less biased after being exposed to children of different races' preferences [Doyle & Aboud, 1995]. Doyle and Aboud [1995, p. 225] explain, 'when children accept the legitimacy of an out-group child's preference, it directly affects their own preferences'.

Similarly, Doyle et al. [1988] found that as children's age increased, cognitive developments such as their ethnic constancy and conservation scores increased. Children's ability to see both positive and negative attributes in in-group and out-group members was related specifically to conservation scores, that is, the child's level of concrete operational thinking. With these cognitive developments, Doyle et al. [1988, p. 15] claim that 'differential attributions of positive and negative traits to one's own and another ethnic group may be the inverse of perceiving the groups as similar'. That is, over time, children may see similarities between themselves and other groups, and this observation of similar attributes may replace bias. Doyle et al. [1988] suggest that this perceived similarity indicates the presence of the ability to understand individuals belonging to a particular group can have different traits, and both positive and negative attributes. Unlike Clark et al. [1980], however, they did not find evidence of a decrease in preference resulting from the child's desire to give socially acceptable answers.

According to Doyle et al. [1988, p. 14], 'older children showed no tendency to conform to the perceptions of the experimenter's attitudes more than young children did'. In fact, social desirability decreased from first to fifth grade. Instead, cognitive development allowing children to recognize similarity is associated with a decrease in prejudice. These findings suggests that White children's cognitive developments lead to a better understanding of racial categories and ability to see positive qualities in individuals despite race. Common in these studies was a decrease in prejudice associated with cognitive developments.

In assessing the relationship between cognitive ability and stereotyped responding in Black children, Averhart and Bigler [1997] found that the more a child developed cognitively with age, particularly with classification skills, the less they gave responses that fell in line with stereotypes. The ideas of more cognitively mature children about racial categories were more flexible with better classification abilities. Despite increasing cognitive ability, in memory tasks in which children were to recall either stereotype-consistent information or stereotype-inconsistent information, children's biases were apparent in that they remembered nonstereotypic information more frequently than they remembered stereotypic information. Averhart and Bigler [1997, p. 381] suggest that memory tasks, unlike the Preschool Racial Attitudes Measure II (PRAM II) questionnaire, are cognitively demanding and '[tap] automatic forms of stereotyping (i.e. bias that is not easily altered)'. The PRAM, on the other hand, may 'permit older children to monitor their responding in [an] attempt to override their biases. In this regard, like some studies with White children [Clark et al., 1980; Doyle et al., 1998], cognitive developments were associated with less-biased responding to test measures, and possibly, an increased ability to provide social desirable answers.

In contrast, Branch and Newcombe [1986] found that as children develop cognitively, their racial attitudes change. Branch and Newcombe [1986] attribute the changes in Black children's preferences with age in part to their cognitive developments: 'One explanation for the apparent change in attitudes with age is that older children are more mature cognitively and have better ability to synthesize their social experiences' [Branch and Newcombe, 1986, p. 719]. In addition, they suggest that with age and cognitive advancement, children will begin to hear and understand the messages they have been taught by family members and other within their social circle. In this regard, cognitive developments in Black children do not just increase their ability to provide socially desirable answers, but give them the ability to process competing ideas.

Similarly, Spencer [1982] found that social and cultural cognitions that increase with age, particularly the development of language, decentration, and race awareness, are related to changes in Black children's racial attitudes. Results from Spencer's [1982] study indicate that there is a progressive understanding of societal color bias by young children. Spencer [1982, p. 81] goes on to explain '. . .it appears clear from empirical findings that definitive links exist between the cognitive and affective domains' and that changes in a child's personal identity (self-concept) and the group identity (racial-attitudes and preferences) occur as a result of 'the child's developing cognitive construction of the world'. Specifically, cognitive developments allow the child's personal identity to be separate from their group identity. This suggests that it is possible that Black children's in-group or out-group feelings and preferences are separate from the growing knowledge of stereotypes that exist in society.

Likewise, Semaj [1980, p. 77] found that cognitive developments in Black children 'improve the child's 'perception of social reality'. As impersonal and social cognitive development increases, there is a qualitative and quantitative change in Black children's social affect to race. Semaj [1980, p. 73] found that for younger children ages 4–7, 'racial evaluation and preference was dependent on the level of social cognitive abilities for racial classification and constancy'. In line with this finding, older children (8–11 years of age) without racial constancy evaluated in-group and out-group members in a way that was similar to the 4- to 7-year-olds. Once the cognitive developments of racial classification and constancy are established, Black children ages 4–7 show consistent ethno-centric preferences for Whites. Cognitive developments facilitate in-group racial evaluation preferences in young children, but facilitate less-biased response in older children 8–11 years of age. Young children without racial constancy were more favorable towards Whites in terms of their racial preferences while older children without constancy show a reverse of this trend [Semaj, 1980, p. 75].

Findings indicate Black children 'are aware of the social norms of de facto racial segregation' [Semaj, 1980, p. 75]. Semaj [1980] explains that these norms are not fully internalized and that 'children can and do differentiate between the (racial) preference for another child (in a photograph) and for self. Racial choices of the self were less definitive than choices for another child, indicating the child perceives race as less important to self than social norms dictate.

Semaj [1980] explains, however, that although children are beginning to 'understand that people are categorized into various ethno-racial groups, they do not yet understand the bases for these groupings', and that they are beginning to 'learn the evaluation of and the connotations associated with these colors [Black and White] in the forms of stereotypes' [p. 76]. He asserts that Black children's ethno-racial evaluation resulting from cognitive developments is simply a 'regurgitation' of the input received from the social environment and is independent of self-evaluations.

In line with Davey and Mullin's [1980, p. 248] conclusion that 'minority group children have little doubt as to who has the favored place in the social pecking order', studies indicate that cognitive developments bring about a social awareness in Black children. These developments and awareness are linked not only to the ability to attribute both positive and negative characteristics to both Blacks and Whites, or the ability to give socially desirable answers. Instead, common in these studies is the idea that cognitive developments impact Black children's affect towards their own and others' racial groups.

Perceived Similarity and Dissimilarity
According to Doyle and Aboud [1995, p. 212], 'it has been established that the perception of similarity within races and dissimilarity between races in an important component of racial prejudice'.

Aboud [1980] found that in both Black and White children there is as stronger perceived in-group perceived similarity and out-group dissimilarity in older children (first graders) versus younger children (preschool aged). While these perceptions increase with age for all children regardless of race, Black and White children differed significantly in out-group dissimilarity measures. 'Black judged fewer out-group charters to be different from them than did Whites' [Aboud, 1980, p. 2]. In addition for Black children, in-group preference, out-group dissimilarity and grade were all factors that influenced out-group attitudes. For Black children, while in-group preference had a negative effect on out-group attitudes, dissimilarity to out-groups was positively related to out-group attitudes. In summary, the more out-group members were perceived as dissimilar to oneself, the more positive one's feelings were towards that group.

Aboud [1980] suggests that self-other differences are accompanied by confidence in one's identity. Aboud [1980] suggests that Black children in this study may have had this confidence given that they attended schools that were predominantly Black in student numbers, teachers, and administration, in a multiethnic, urban community: 'If social comparison within one's community is indeed the mechanism by which children evaluate themselves and others [. . .] these children would attach a positive value to being Black' [Aboud, 1980, p. 205]. In addition, Aboud [1980] postulates that such a diverse community such as Montreal could have been responsible, in part, for these positive feelings in these minority children, instead of the 'usual preference for Whites' [p. 205].

For White children, on the other hand, only in-group preference predicted out-group attitudes in that the more they preferred their in-group, the more negative they felt towards out-group members: 'White children's attitudes were unrelated to dissimilarity' [p. 204]. According to Aboud [1980, p. 207], 'Whites have always been encouraged to distinguish between themselves and ethnic minorities' and 'this popular belief is borne out by the data: Blacks perceived fewer differences than did Whites who were already close to ceiling level in preschool'.

Prejudice was associated with 'perception of more similarity between races and less similarity within a race'. Counter-bias was associated with 'perception of less similarity between races and greater acceptance of racial differences in preference' [p. 222]. Specifically, perceptions of between-race similarity was related to decreases in prejudice and in increase in counter-bias (more positive attributes given to out-group members and more negative evaluations towards their own in-group). Doyle et al. [1988] found that 'perceived similarity [also] seems to reflect an ability to hold differentiated perceptions of groups', that is, that individuals within the groups may possess different traits.

In addition, Doyle and Aboud [1995] found that White children perceived more similarity within and between races, as they got older. Perceptions of within-race similarity were associated with racial attitudes, specifically higher out-group prejudice. This was found to be stable across age (in kindergarteners to third graders). According to

Doyle and Aboud [1995, p. 226], '. . .perceptual differentiation within race is an important individual difference relevant to prejudice, even in young children'.

In summary, while perceived out-group dissimilarity predicted positive in-group feelings in Black children, White children's attitudes were unrelated to dissimilarity. For White children, perceived between race as well as within-race similarity was associated with out-group prejudice. Between-race dissimilarity was associated with counter-bias.

Preference and Identification

In the studies presented, Black and White children differed in their patterns of concordance, that is, in same race identification and preference. Davey and Mullin [1980, p. 247] found that in their sample of 512 children, 'overall some 63% of the children present a concordant pattern, mainly by expressing an own group choice on both the identification and preference tests'. Results revealed that boys were more consistent in showing these patterns than girls. Likewise, results showed that it is very unlikely that a child will make two out-group choices, thus completely rejecting their in-group. White children were found to have higher levels of concordance, however, than Black children. Forty percent of Black children were found to have an in-group identification accompanied by an out-group preference.

Preference and Race Awareness

Spencer [1984] found that racial awareness in Black children was positively and significantly correlated with White bias or White preference. That is, the more a Black child was aware of racial differences, the more they preferred Whites to their in-group. In fact, Spencer [1984] indicates that race awareness was the single significant predictor of pro-White attitudes in Black children. Specifically, younger preschool children were found to be as equally biased as older kindergarten children [Spencer, 1984]. In addition,

girls' racial majority-preference attitudes were significantly and positively correlated with their racial awareness. Overall, children who scored higher on measures of self-awareness were more White-oriented in their preferences that children who were in the 'task failure' group, that is, not as aware of race [p. 438]. For younger girls (between the ages of 4 and 4.7 years), and boys (between the ages of 5.7 and 6.5 years), as these White-preferenced attitudes increased, self-concept decreased. According to Spencer [1984, p. 440], it appears that Black 'children are able to conceptualize and compartmentalize a view of self which is independent of attitudes surrounding the evaluation of their racial group'. No studies presented indicate that White children's racial awareness was as correlated with strong out-group feelings.

Research Question #2b: How do Black and White Children Differ in the Development of Personal Stereotypes and Stereotype Consciousness?

Inferring Personal Stereotypes

Although McKown and Weinstein [2003] found that the ability to infer another's stereotype precedes the awareness of broadly held stereotypes, no differences were found between Black and White children in the development of the ability to infer an individual's stereotype. Ninety-three% of all children in the study, regardless of gender and age, were found to be able to infer another individual's stereotypes by age 10.

Broadly Held Stereotypes

According to McKown and Weinstein [2003], where Black and White children differ is in their awareness of broadly held stereotypes. Findings indicate that 'a greater proportion of children from stigmatized groups [Blacks and Latinos] are aware of broadly held stereotypes' [p. 506] compared to White (and Asian) children, who are not members of stigmatized groups. Children from stigmatized ethnic groups also had an earlier awareness of broadly held stereotypes compared to children from non-stigmatized groups. As noted earlier, at age 6, 15% of minority children from stigmatized groups were aware of broadly held stereotypes. Only 7% of children from nonstigmatized groups were aware of broadly held stereotypes by the age of 6. Similarly, by age 10, 80% of Black (and Latino) children versus 63% of White (and Asian) children were aware of broadly held stereotypes. According to McKown and Weinstein [2003, p. 506], the fact that '. . .children from stigmatized groups were more likely to be aware of broadly held stereotypes probably reflects the greater salience of stereotypes in the daily life of children from stigmatized groups'. The authors further explain that '. . .ethnic minority children's development is partly shaped by the experience of minority status' [McKown & Weinstein, 2003, p. 506].

Research Question #3: What Are the Consequences Related to the Development of Personal Stereotypes and Stereotype Consciousness in Black and White Children?
Findings from Spencer [1982] indicated a link between identity related variables and cognitive performance measures. Specifically, Spencer [1982] found that for children with lower socioeconomic statuses, the shift in preference from White bias to a more Afrocentric orientation resulted in decreased performance on standardized tests measuring language. This standardized measure, the McCarthy Index, assesses both receptive and expressive language. By age nine, lower income children's bias begins to level so that their scores indicate no racial preference, although children's orientations have become more Afrocentric. According to Spencer [1984, p. 80], 'this lack of definite Afrocentric orientation for attitudes and preferences is associated with a decline in performance on [the] standardized measure'.

The consequences of the development of stereotype consciousness are also academic in nature, and can adversely impact test performance. McKown and Weinstein [2003] examined the relationship between broadly held stereotypes and cognitive task performance. The first cognitive tasks included writing as many letters of the alphabet as possible in 45 s from the letter Z backwards. This cognitive task focused heavily on working memory and concentration, both being sensitive to anxiety. The researchers found that 'among children from stigmatized ethnic groups aware of broadly held stereotypes, on 1 of the 2 challenging cognitive tasks and self-reported effort, diagnostic testing conditions led to stereotype threat effects. The main hypothesis was confirmed in that when children from stigmatized groups became aware of broadly held stereotypes, this awareness indirectly activated Stereotype Threat that significantly hampered cognitive performance. According to the researchers, stereotype threat theory posits 'others' stereotypes are threatening and hamper performance when situations induce targets to become concerned that others will judge their performance stereotypically' [McKown and Weinstein, p. 510]. In this regard 'Awareness of others' stereotypes is necessary for individually activated stereotypes to be activated threatening and affect performance' [McKown and Weinstein, p. 510].

Black and White children differ in that indirectly activated stereotypes only adversely affect the performance of children from academically stigmatized ethnic groups (Black children) who are aware of broadly held stereotypes. McKown and Weinstein [2003] found no consequences of decreased test performance related to White children's awareness of broadly held stereotypes.

Neither age nor ability to infer one's stereotypes predicts response to stereotype threat conditions. Instead, '. . .knowing about broadly held stereotypes opens the possibility that children from stigmatized groups will be concerned (about) being judged on the basis of those stereotypes, a possibility that can lead to self-fulfilling prophecy' [McKown and Weinstein, p. 510]. Given their findings, McKown and Weinstein [2003] show the effects of stereotype threat become salient for a large number of children of color by the third grade.

Importantly, some children had this awareness as early as age 6, which has consequences given that high-stakes standardized testing is now taking place. Testing conditions that elicit stereotype threat conditions and negatively impact the academic performance of children of color can start in elementary school and differentially impact children's academic outcomes, thus placing Black children on tracks that would threaten their future academic success.

Finally, McKown and Weinstein [2003] found that stereotype threat conditions led to greater levels of self-reported effort withdrawal. In this regard, stereotype threat effects brought on by awareness of broadly held stereotypes can not only impact academic performance in Black children, but can possibly cause these children to disengage from academic domains altogether.

Conclusions

Over the last 30 years, little research has been done to understand the development of stereotypes in Black and White children. Although definitive statements cannot be made based on the limited amount of literature, there are some general conclusions with regard to the three research questions.

With regard to the development of stereotypes, Black and White children can have racial preferences as early as 4 and 5 years old. Although most children's differential preferences for in-group or out-group decrease with time, White children generally tend to be more consistent in their positive evaluations and preferences of their in-group compared to Black children. White children also exhibit greater patterns of concordance, that is, greater in-group identification and in-group preference. With increasing age, Black and White children learn to evaluate individuals of both races positively, that is, they are able to recognize positive characteristics in individuals that may run counter to early biases they exhibited.

Findings indicate that White children's prejudices decrease over time, that is, that they gain more positive attitudes towards Black children as they mature; yet they still maintain more positive in-group feelings. In contrast, Black children's out-group preference and in-group attitudes were found to fluctuate, but remain higher for Whites than their in-group.

Cognitive development in Black and White children was associated with an ability to evaluate racial groups more critically, attributing positive and negative characteristics to both groups. Some researchers explored the possibility that, with cognitive maturation, it was possible that older children were able to give more socially desirable responses. Decreases in prejudice, then, may have resulted from the children's growing ability to understand social categories and therefore respond accordingly, particularly in White children. Likewise, cognitive developments in Black children also resulted in better understanding of the social meanings behind concepts of 'Black' and 'White'. The fact that findings indicted a greater awareness, but responses that favored White individuals, suggests that Black children's cognitive development resulted in affective changes in their preferences, not simply a desire to provide socially acceptable answers in the presence of the test administrator.

In Black and White children, perceived similarity and dissimilarity between and within races impacted children's preferences and attitudes towards in-group and out-group members. Race awareness was another factor attributed to differences in the developmental trajectories of Black and White children. Among Black children, greater racial awareness leads to increased White preference, a pattern not found in studies with White children.

Black and White children were found to differ significantly in the development of stereotype consciousness. By age 10, almost all children could infer another individual's stereotype. Black children, who were identified as being academically stigmatized, showed an earlier and greater awareness of broadly held stereotypes than White children. Academic consequences, particularly decreased performance due to stereotype threat, were found only for the minority status (Black) children. Stereotype threat conditions led Black children who were aware of broadly held stereotypes, to experience a decrease in performance on cognitive tasks and to report higher levels of effort withdrawals. Both could cause the children to further disidentify with academic domains, thus contributing to the racial achievement gap.

The development of stereotypes in Black and White children, though similar in many ways, seems to only hold dire academic consequences for Black children. Black children are disproportionately impacted by stereotypes in academic domains due to their stigmatized status. As children become more aware of the social meanings behind racial categories and gain an awareness of broadly held stereotypes, they begin to not only evaluate their own groups less positively and express a pro-White bias, but they also disproportionally experience decrements in performance under the fear of confirming negative stereotypes about their racial group. While the development of stereotypes is a natural process in which all children take part in order to help them understand concepts related to racial differences, it may be Black children's introduction to societal racism.

Limitations and Future Directions

Many studies used forced-choice techniques, which make the child pick between Black and White in order to evaluate their racial attitudes.

Possibly, pro-racial attitudes, particularly for one's in-group, may be weaker when evaluated in a way that does not force the child to think of their racial group in relation to another. More studies implementing multiple measures are needed in order to gain a more holistic understanding of the development of children's racial attitudes.

In addition, many of the studies presented were cross-sectional. Patterns found among groups of students and changes across age may not reflect developmental patterns as much as they could result from cohort effects. Longitudinal studies exploring the development of racial stereotypes in children are needed to eliminate the possibility of cohort effects and help give insight to actual age-related developmental changes in children.

Further, only two studies attempted to examine the consequences of stereotype development in children. Given that Black children are disproportionally impacted by negative racial stereotypes (and stereotype threat), and that they hold a stigmatized status in academic domains, it is important that more studies draw connections between the development and consequences of racial stereotypes for the creation of meaningful interventions.

Finally, the results of the study may not be generalizable to Black children's worldviews outside of the United States (or even biracial children within the United States). Further research is needed to draw conclusions regarding the impact of stereotypes on Black and White children in countries where the history of prejudice, and the history of institutional racism, differ from that of the United States.

References

*Aboud, F.E. (1980). A test of ethnocentrism with young children. *Canadian Journal of Behavioural Science / Revue canadienne des sciences du comportement, 12,* 195–209.

Aboud, F.E., & Skerry, S. (1984). The development of ethnic attitudes: A critical review. *Journal of Cross-Cultural Psychology, 15,* 3–34.

Ashmore, R.D., & Del Boca, E.K. (1981). Conceptual approaches to stereotypes and stereotyping. In D.L. Hamilton (Ed.), *Cognitive processes in stereotyping and intergroup behavior* (pp. 1–35). Hillsdale: Erlbaum.

*Averhart, C.J., & Bigler, R.S. (1997). Shades of meaning: Skin tone, racial attitudes, and constructive memory in African-American children. *Journal of Experimental Child Psychology, 67,* 363–388.

*Branch, C.W., & Newcombe, N. (1986). Racial attitude development among young Black children as a function of parental attitudes: A longitudinal and cross-sectional study. *Child Development, 57,* 712–721.

*Bigler, R.S., & Liben, L.S. (1993). A cognitive-developmental approach to racial stereotyping and constructive memory in Euro-American children. *Child Development, 64,* 1507–1518.

*Clark, A., Hocevar, D., & Dembo, M.H. (1980). The role of cognitive development in children's explanations and preference of skin color. *Developmental Psychology, 16,* 332–339.

Clark, K.B., & Clark, M.K. (1939). The development of consciousness of self and the emergence of racial identification in Negro preschool children. *Journal of Social Psychology, 10,* 591–599.

Clark, K.B., & Clark, M.K. (1940). Skin color as a factor in racial identification of Negro preschool children. *Journal of Social Psychology, 11,* 159–169.

Crocker, J., & Quinn, D.M. (2000). Social stigma and the self: Meaning, situations, and self-esteem. In T.F. Heatherton, R.E. Kleck, M.R. Hebl & J.G. Hull (Eds.), *The social psychology of stigma* (pp. 153–183). New York: Guilford Press.

*Davey, A.G., & Mullin, P.N. (1980). Ethnic identification and preference of British primary school children. *Journal of Child Psychology and Psychiatry, 21,* 241–251.

*Doyle, A.B., & Aboud, F.E. (1995). A longitudinal study of White children's racial prejudice as a social-cognitive development. *Merrill-Palmer Quarterly, 41,* 209–228.

*Doyle, A.B., Beaudet, J., & Aboud, F.E. (1988). Developmental patterns in the flexibility of children's ethnic attitudes. *Journal of Cross-Cultural Psychology, 19,* 3–18.

McGarty, C., Yzerbyt, V.Y., & Spears, R. (2002). *Stereotypes as explanations: The formation of meaningful beliefs about social groups.* New York: Cambridge University Press.

*McKown, C., & Weinstein, R. (2003). The development and consequences of stereotype-consciousness in childhood. *Child Development, 74,* 498–515.

*Semaj, L. (1980). The development of racial evaluation and preference: A cognitive approach. *Journal of Black Psychology, 6,* 59–79.

Slaughter-Defoe, D.T., Johnson, D.J., & Spencer, M.B. (2009). Race and children's development. In R.A. Shweder, T.R. Bidell, A.C. Dailey, S.D. Dixon, P.J. Miller & J. Modell (Eds.), *The child: An encyclopedic companion* (pp. 801–805). Chicago: University of Chicago Press.

*Spencer, M.B. (1982). Personal and group identity of Black children: An alternative synthesis. *Genetic Psychology Monographs, 103,* 59–84.

*Spencer, M.B. (1984). Black children's race awareness, racial attitudes, and self-concept: A reinterpretation. *Journal of Child Psychology and Psychiatry, 25,* 433–441.

Steele, C.M., & Aronson, J. (1995). Stereotype threat and the intellectual test performance of African-Americans. *Journal of Personality and Social Psychology, 69,* 797–811.

*Williams, L., & Davidson, D. (2009). Interracial and intra-racial stereotypes and constructive memory in 7- and 9-year-old African American children. *Journal of Applied Developmental Psychology, 30,* 336–377.

*Zinser, O., Rich, M.C., & Bailey, R.C. (1981). Sharing behavior and racial preference in children. *Motivation and Emotion, 5,* 619–629.

*Designates one of 14 identified studies in References.

Ms. Erin D. Bogan (MA 2010, Applied Psychology and Human Development, University of Pennsylvania) graduated magna cum laude from the University of California Berkeley with Bachelor degrees in English and Social Welfare. She then studied at the University of Pennsylvania where she received her Masters degree. Offered admission to several doctoral programs, she chose to enroll in fall 2011 at the University of Michigan, Ann Arbor for PhD studies. She plans continued study of the impact of stigma on the achievement and social well-being of students of color.

Dr. Diana T. Slaughter-Defoe (PhD 1968, University of Chicago) received her doctorate from the Committee on Human Development in developmental and clinical psychology, and is presently the Constance E. Clayton Professor Emerita in the Graduate School of Education at the University of Pennsylvania. Her research interests have included culture, primary education, and home-school relations facilitating in-school academic achievement. Since retirement, she has also edited: *Black Educational Choice: Assessing the Private and Public Alternatives to K-12 Public Schools* [Praeger, 2011] with colleagues, and *Messages for Educational Leadership: The Constance E. Clayton Lectures, 1998–2007* [Peter Lang Publishers, 2012]. She is presently writing a memoir about her career that spanned 40-plus years in academia and higher education.

Prof. Diana T. Slaughter-Defoe
Graduate School of Education
The University of Pennsylvania
3700 Walnut Street
Philadelphia, PA 19104–6216 (USA)
Tel. +1 215 582 7036
E-Mail dianasd@gse.upenn.edu

Commentary

Slaughter-Defoe DT (ed): Racial Stereotyping and Child Development.
Contrib Hum Dev. Basel, Karger, 2012, vol 25, pp 20–23

Should Stereotype Consciousness Be Taught to Children? A Discussion Informed by Bogan and Slaughter-Defoe's Through the Eyes of a Child

Commentary on Bogan and Slaughter-Defoe

Rebecca S. Bigler · Yamanda Wright

University of Texas at Austin, Austin, Tex., USA

Consistent with Bogan and Slaughter-Defoe, as well as other scholars [e.g., Garcia Coll & Vázquez García, 1995], we believe that race has a pervasive influence on human development. The United States of America, for example, is characterized by persistent disparities between Black and White children in the domains of mental well-being, physical health, and academic achievement. Racial segregation of schools and neighborhoods is also still prevalent [Orfield, 2001] and, as Bogan and Slaughter-Defoe's review indicates, racial stereotyping persists even among very young children.

While all children are affected by race-related attitudes, children often have little meta-cognitive awareness of the influence of race on human development. One such form of knowledge addressed by Bogan and Slaughter-Defoe is racial stereotype consciousness (i.e., awareness that others endorse racial stereotypes). Moreover, a controversial issue related to children's understanding of the effects of racial attitudes is whether young children should be taught stereotype consciousness explicitly. Should adults intentionally make children aware of racial stereotypes? Should children be taught about historical and contemporary cases of racial bias? If so, at which age should these concepts be introduced and with what degree of depth and detail? And should discussion of these concepts be framed equivalently or differently for children who are oppressed versus privileged by racial biases?

The degree to which these issues are contested was made clear to us when the journal *Child Development* published an intervention in which elementary school-age White children were taught history lessons that included explicit discussion of racial discrimination [Hughes, Bigler, & Levy, 2007]. Some individuals decried the work as unethical and immoral, arguing that the lessons had induced young White children to feel negatively about themselves because of practices associated with their racial in-group but over which they had no control and in which they did not participate. Overall, we believe that stereotype consciousness is an important component of understanding the social world and an appropriate topic of instruction for elementary school-age children. Nonetheless, we feel that it is important to consider – and explore empirically – the potential risks and benefits of teaching children about racial stereotypes.

In our commentary, we evaluate arguments concerning whether to teach stereotype consciousness to children. Drawing on Bogan and Slaughter-Defoe's review, we discuss the potential risks and benefits associated with stereotype consciousness in early childhood, ultimately making the claim that carefully designed lessons about stereotyping and prejudice would be advantageous to young children. Our aim is to inspire additional theoretical and empirical work on children's racial knowledge and attitudes with the goal of identifying the best possible practices for raising children who celebrate diversity, promote social justice, and thrive socially, emotionally, and academically.

Does Teaching about Racial Stereotypes Induce Awareness of Race?

One argument against presenting young children with information about racial stereotypes is that addressing the topic will provoke race-based thinking among children who do not yet 'notice' race. In other words, children who do not see the world as divided into racial categories will be sparked to categorize people as 'Black' and 'White' by the introduction of lessons about racial stereotypes.

Although many laypeople continue to believe that young children do not notice race, research indicates that children begin to attend to race during infancy. Newborn infants, for example, demonstrate no spontaneous preference for faces from their own ethnic group; however, when shown own-race faces paired with other-race faces, 3-month-old infants show a significant looking preference for own-race faces [Kelly et al., 2005]. The effect has been found among Caucasian, African, and Chinese infants [Bar-Haim, Ziv, Lamy & Hodes, 2006; Kelly, et al., 2009; Kelly et al., 2005]. Furthermore, children show a pattern of responding to individual faces of each race that suggests that they become 'experts' in the area of racial recognition of faces during infancy [Quinn et al.,

2011]. In summary, very young children spontaneously use race as a basis for categorizing others, and thus discussing racial stereotypes is highly unlikely to cause children to begin to attend to race.

Does Teaching about Racial Stereotypes Lead to Endorsement of Racial Stereotypes?

A second argument for protecting children from exposure to information about racial stereotypes is that addressing the topic will lead to personal endorsement of those stereotypes. So, for example, introducing children to the notion that Whites have historically viewed Blacks as intellectually inferior might lead children to endorse such views themselves.

Importantly, Bogan and Slaughter-Defoe's review makes clear that Black and White preschoolers show Eurocentric biases when responding to questions regarding color, peer preferences, and traits of hypothetical characters at very early ages. Young children are not only aware of race, but they appear to have internalized the status differences between the races, and thus view Whites more favorably than Blacks. It is highly unlikely, then, that discussing racial stereotypes will cause the *onset* of racial stereotyping.

Although informing children about racial stereotypes is unlikely to cause racial stereotyping, it is possible that such information might facilitate stereotyping among those who are already biased. There is a tendency for individuals to justify the status quo and thus it seems possible that children who learn that Whites have long viewed Blacks as, for example, dishonest might come to believe that this particular view is accurate. Hughes et al. [2007] tested this hypothesis by examining the effects of learning about historical racism on Black and White children's racial attitudes. Their results showed that exposure to information about historical racism improved White children's attitudes about Black people and left views of Whites unaffected. The lessons failed to affect Black children's attitudes towards Whites or Blacks. Thus, it appears that learning that other individuals endorse racial biases does not necessarily lead children to internalize or emulate such views.

Are Young Children Too Cognitively Immature to Understand Racial Stereotypes?

A third argument for restricting children's exposure to information about racial stereotypes is that children are too cognitively immature to grasp concepts integral to a complete, adult-like comprehension of racial bias. It is possible that understanding racism requires cognitive abilities, such as perspective taking or multiple classification skill, that are beyond the intellectual scope of young children, and thus teaching stereotype consciousness to young children may be ineffective or even counterproductive.

As Bogan and Slaughter-Defoe note, children become aware of others' racial biases by age 6. Thus, children typically personally endorse and recognize racial stereotypes before they have a full understanding of the concept. However, there is evidence that moral reasoning emerges and is applied to intergroup attitudes early in development [Killen & Stangor, 2001]. Together these findings suggest that school-age children have a strong sense of fairness that could be leveraged by lessons emphasizing the moral implications of racial bias (e.g., inequity), even if they are incapable of understanding the nuances of sophisticated psychological constructs such as racial stereotyping. Future work should examine more closely children's developing views of social stereotyping and prejudice.

Does Learning about Racial Stereotypes Induce Negative Affect?

An additional argument for avoidance of the topic of stereotype consciousness with children is that Black children may feel victimized, experience hopelessness, or resent Whites as a result of such information. It is also possible that White children will feel guilty or become defensive in light of their new stereotype consciousness. The notion that children should be protected from potentially upsetting information about the world is intuitively appealing. In the intervention described earlier, Hughes et al. [2007] examined the effects of learning about historical racism on Black and White children's racial attitudes. The authors note that levels of guilt and defensiveness were elevated among some White students who had learned about racism, but remained at very low levels. Furthermore, levels of anger among Black students were unaffected by the lessons. It will be important for future work to follow-up this initial evidence that learning about racial stereotyping is not necessarily emotionally harmful with alternative forms of lesson content.

Does Learning about Racial Stereotypes Undermine Cognitive Performance?

Stereotype consciousness may affect children's achievement in school. As Bogan and Slaughter-Defoe discuss in their conclusion, stereotype threat conditions lead to impaired performance on cognitive tasks and greater levels of self-reported effort withdrawal. Although it seems possible the teaching children about racial stereotypes may increase stigmatized children's vulnerability to stereotype threat, stereotype threat effects are not inevitable. Social psychologists have begun to identify conditions (e.g., testing conditions and instructions) that prevent the operation of stereotype threat [Davies, Spencer & Steele, 2005; Johns, Schmader & Martens, 2005; Marx & Roman, 2002]. Because racial stereotype consciousness inevitably develops during childhood, the best strategy may be to develop lessons that both introduce children to the concept of racial stereotypes and, simultaneously, to strategies that will prevent such knowledge from undermining their own goals and performance.

Conclusions and Future Directions for Research

Overall, there is much left to learn about the formation, function, and consequences of stereotype consciousness in childhood. General discomfort about discussing issues of race and racial prejudice with children has resulted in a dearth of knowledge about the most effective ways to convey such information. Yet ethics dictate that educators provide children with information about the role of race in shaping human lives and relationships. Without intervention, children receive very little information about race that might counteract their own developing biases as they observe racial inequalities in the world around them. We believe that the process of informing children about the effects of racial attitudes should begin in elementary school, and furthermore, that the potential positive outcomes outweigh the potential negative outcomes associated with such learning. As with adults, we believe that teaching stereotype consciousness to young children has the potential to improve racial attitudes and race relations.

References

Bar-Haim, Y., Ziv, T., Lamy, D., & Hodes, R.M. (2006). Nature and nurture in own-race face processing. *Psychological Science, 17,* 159–163.

Davies, P.G., Spencer, S.J., & Steele, C.M. (2005). Clearing the air: Identity safety moderates the effects of stereotype threat on women's leadership aspirations. *Journal of Personality and Social Psychology, 88,* 276–287.

García Coll, C.T., & Vázquez García, H.A. (1995). Developmental processes and their influence on interethnic and interracial relations. In W.B. Hawley & A. Jackson (Eds.), *Toward a common destiny: Improving race and ethnic relations in America* (pp. 103–130). San Francisco: Jossey-Bass.

Hughes, J.M., Bigler, R.S., & Levy, S.R. (2007). Consequences of learning about historical racism among European American and African American children. *Child Development, 78,* 1689–1705.

Johns, M., Schmader, T., & Martens, A. (2005). Knowing is half the battle: Teaching stereotype threat as a means of improving women's math performance. *Psychological Science, 16,* 175–179.

Kelly, D.J., Liu, S., Lee, K., Quinn, P.C., Pascalis, O., Slater, A.M., & Ge, L. (2009). Development of the other-race effect in infancy: Evidence towards universality? *Journal of Experimental Child Psychology, 104,* 105–114.

Kelly, D.J., Quinn, P.C., Slater, A.M., Lee, K., Gibson, A., Smith, M., & Pascalis, O. (2005). Three-month-olds, but not newborns, prefer own-race faces. *Developmental Science, 8,* 31–36.

Killen, M., & Stangor, C. (2001). Children's social reasoning about inclusion and exclusion in gender and race peer group contexts. *Child Development, 72,* 174–186.

Marx, D.M., & Roman, J.S. (2002). Female role models: Protecting women's math test performance. *Personality and Social Psychology Bulletin, 28,* 1183–1193.

Orfield, G. (2001). Schools more separate: Consequences of a decade of resegregation. Cambridge, MA: The Civil Rights Project, Harvard University.

Quinn, P.C., Anzures, G., Izard, C.E., Lee, K., Pascalis, O., Slater, A.M., & Tanaka, J.W. (2011). Looking across domains to understand infant representation of emotion. *Emotion Review, 3,* 197–206.

Dr. Rebecca S. Bigler (PhD 1991, Department of Psychology, The Pennsylvania State University) is Professor of Psychology and Women's and Gender Studies at the University of Texas at Austin. She studies the causes and consequences of social stereotyping and prejudice among children, with a particular focus on gender and racial attitudes. She has also worked to develop and test intervention strategies aimed at reducing children's social stereotyping and intergroup biases. Her work has appeared in top journals in the field of developmental psychology (*Monographs of the Society for Research in Child Development, Developmental Psychology*), and has been covered by major media outlets (*Newsweek, NBC Dateline, New York Times*). Her research has been supported by Teaching Tolerance and the National Science Foundation.

Ms. Yamanda Wright (BA 2007, Stanford University) is a doctoral student in the Department of Psychology at the University of Texas at Austin. Her research interests include the effects of social identities and attitudes on children's social relationships, information processing, and academic outcomes. Her master's thesis examined the effect of an experimental manipulation aimed at improving cross-race student-teacher relationships on kindergartners' adjustment to the school environment.

Rebecca S. Bigler
Department of Psychology
1 University Station A8000
University of Texas at Austin
Austin, TX 78712 (USA)
E-Mail bigler@psy.utexas.edu

Slaughter-Defoe DT (ed): Racial Stereotyping and Child Development.
Contrib Hum Dev. Basel, Karger, 2012, vol 25, pp 24–27

What's Not in the Box?: Historical and Population Change as Contextual Features in the Study of Race-Based Development of Children

Commentary on Bogan and Slaughter-Defoe

Deborah J. Johnson

Department of Human Development and Family Studies, Michigan State University, East Lansing, Mich., USA

The Bogan and Slaughter-Defoe chapter provides much material for our consideration and refinement of race based constructs associated with race preference, salience and identity. Reading the chapter raised many issues for me, and I found myself thinking about how rarely we raise the broader issues of context in this field. In particular, I intend to address, in brief, three points (a) social historical context, (b) demographic change and shift, both of which are related to the (c) rise and change in racial-ethnic labels and meaning, such as biraciality/multiraciality. These issues of context and their relation to identity development, race-based socialization, and attitudes remain underexplored.

Social Historical Context

It is interesting that this review of the literature on African-American and Euro-American children's racial identity, preferences, and stereotyping takes place in this historical moment in time and covers the period from 1980 to 2010. In the last 30 years or so, there have been many additional studies of these constructs added to the literature, particularly with respect to stereotyping and processes that surround preference and prejudice in children. Moreover, the science around the study of these constructs, identity, race preference and prejudice is stronger. This period is worthy of being marked not only for the extension of its core constructs concerning race and prejudice in children but also for the enhancement of methodological and analytical approaches in these studies. Another important factor to consider is the historical moment in which these findings reside and the critical evolution of the contributions made.

In the research conducted during the 20–30 years preceding 1980, Black children and families were largely newly integrated into urban schools and communities, many having migrated from Southern towns and cities in the 1940s to 1970s to the more lucrative industries of Northern regions during the Second Great Migration [Alexander, 1998; Hahn, 2003]. National, municipal, and school level educational policies had, in many instances, been legislatively arranged into compensatory programs and regulations to overcome the Jim Crow exclusions and imbalances of previous historical times. Social change, research on identity and prejudice in children, and educational policy were linked via a variety of examples. The most notable among those examples, of course, was the 1954 Brown vs. The Board of Education decision where the earlier Clark and Clark studies were critical sources of information for the argument, resulting in mandated school desegregation [Bergner, 2009; Spencer, 2008].

In addition, the civil rights and Black power movements (1950/1960–1980), as well as movements toward greater equality and empowerment for women [Freedom, 1973] marked the era just adjacent to the beginning of the focal period of this chapter and provide the foundation for advances and understandings made from the 1980's to the present. So the findings emphasized in the chapter, come on the heels of these changes and perspectives and have shown variability in race preference, racial identity, and racial attitudes in relation to historical changes and other contextual factors [Brown & Lesane-Brown, 2006; Hraba & Grant, 1970; Thornton, Chatters, Taylor & Allen, 1990]. For example, historical context was very important in a study using three generations of adult children interviewed in the National Survey of Black Americans [Brown & Lesane-Brown, 2006; Jackson, 1991]. The study found that the Great Depression and the economic context informed the messages that parents provided and that children carried forward into their adult lives. In the next generation, changes in migration and the new context of living as well as desegregation experiences were also changing messages about managing and coping with race and racial discrimination. In a study of young children assessed at the height of the Black power movement [Hraba & Grant, 1970], researchers found that positive in-group scores were higher and negative out-group were also higher among children in an all-Black Pan-African school setting than in previous studies. Outside of this specific context and historical period negative out-group scores of Black children were considerably lower.

The situational nature of identity and race-based socialization messages emphasize the importance of context in studies focusing on such variables. Context is a critical element in these researches and is sometimes positioned as if the science and the comparisons are the only varying elements and as such contextual factors, like historical moment, recede in the discussion.

Demographic Change

The period addressed by Bogan and Slaughter-Defoe also sits against a historical backdrop in which a series of significant demographic and educationally relevant changes have occurred that are rarely discussed in this literature. Just prior to the period of the chapter, in the 1970's, the size of the African-American population was peaking in growth. In the period in question the distribution of the American population has shifted, and is shifting again. In current and future trends, Latinos have now exceeded African-Americans in population growth and Euro-Americans will soon become a numerical minority in relation to all peoples of color within the US [US Census Bureau, 2010]. This is a new historical fact and one that will surely affect stereotypes and the experience of racial prejudice among White children and perhaps African American children as well. Another intricacy of population change and growth is the unacknowledged mosaic of the 'African-American' population. This group is now, more than ever, first generation Caribbean-American and 'African'-American (Nigerians, Kenyans, Cameroonians, Sudanese, Ethiopians, South Africans, etc.). This growth is rapid in educational and work settings, and often goes undetected among these many first generation newcomers and second generation descendants. However, the vastly different development of racial attitudes and socialization processes around culture, identity and coping with prejudice [Hughes et al., 2008; Yoshikawa, 2011] make these variations significant in their underrepresentation, particularly in developmental literature. In the future, African-American populations must be better differentiated from the vantage point of multiple ethnicities' in-group descriptions and in analyses.

Shifts in the Meanings of Racial Labels

Multiracial and biracial children are an understudied population in these areas but represent yet another context of meaning in which labels are continuing to shift. If we place the labels and meaning of biracial people in historical context, we would find that there have been longstanding shifts during times of war, changing demographics, and societal perspectives in the last 100 years [Slaughter, Johnson & Spencer, 2009] that would easily map onto the historical discussion of my earlier comments. Most importantly, the shifts in labeling correspond to shifts in moving from the utility of the labels to serve society or political agendas, resulting from imposed agendas around race, miscegenation laws or other political contexts, to the service of individual identities and self-actualization, reflecting greater personal control and fewer consequences associated with that acknowledgement.

Current scholarship on biracial children shows differential processes for identity development and race awareness among this group. In the research, race awareness and affect toward race are informed by children's initial perspectives on racial self-perceptions [Johnson, 1992a] early in a child's life. Parental messages defining identity have some influence, as do obvious racial features. Challenge, 'confusion', and then clarity are likely to be at the core of many cycles in the identity development of biracial children. This is particularly true among those who are of African-American and European-American descent. Developmental period and context are significant in determining what the challenges will be. Assessing the pathways to a comfortable identity will appear as confusion while youth weigh friendship, loyalty, family messages and social cognitions about their race [Johnson, 1992a, b]. Clarity occurs when the important aspects of context, experience with race and negotiating borders, as well as parental message about race emerge as central. Clarity will reign for a time and then new challenges will bring forth new cycles to journey through. These complexities in development are not currently accounted for very easily in a literature that emphasizes monoracial identity processes [Slaughter-Defoe, Johnson & Spencer, 2009].

References

Alexander, J.T. (1998). The Great Migration in comparative perspective: Interpreting the urban origins of Southern Black migrants from Depression era to Pittsburgh. *Social Science History, 22,* Special Issue: Migration and the Labor Markets, pp. 349–376.

Bergner, G. (2009). Black children, White preference: Brown v. Board, the doll tests, and the politics of self-esteem. *American Quarterly, 61,* 299–332.

Brown, T., & Lesane-Brown, C. (2006). Racial socialization message across time. *Social Psychology Quarterly, 69,* 201–213.

Freedom, J. (1973). The origins of the women's liberation movement. *Journal of American Sociology, 78,* 792–811.

Hahn, S. (2003). A nation under our feet: Black political struggles in the rural South, from slavery to the great migration. Cambridge, MA: Harvard University Press.

Hraba, J., & Grant, G. (1970). Black is beautiful: A reexamination of racial preference and identification. *Journal of Personality and Social Psychology, 16,* 398–402.

Hughes, D., Rivas, D., Foust, M., Hagelskamp, C., Gersick, S., & Way, N. (2008). How to catch a moonbeam: A mixed methods approach to ethnic socialization processes among ethnically diverse families. In S. Quintana & C. McKown (Eds.), *Handbook of race, racism, and the developing child* (pp. 226–277). Hoboken: John Wiley and Sons, Inc.

Jackson, J.S. (Ed.) (1991). *Life in Black America.* Newbury Park: Sage Publications.

Johnson, D.J. (1992a). Developmental pathways: Toward an ecological theoretical formulation of race identity in Black/White biracial children. In M.P. Root (Ed.), *Racially mixed people in America: Within, between and beyond* (pp. 37–49). Beverly Hills: Sage Publications.

Johnson, D.J. (1992b). Racial preference and biculturality in biracial preschoolers. *Merrill-Palmer Quarterly, 38,* 233–244.

Slaughter-Defoe, D., Johnson, D.J., & Spencer, M. (2009). Race and children's development. In R.A. Schweder, T.R. Bidell, A.C. Dailey, S.D. Dixon, P.J. Miller & J. Modell (Eds.), *The child: An encyclopedic companion* (pp. 801–806). Chicago: University of Chicago Press.

Spencer, M.B. (2008). Lessons learned and opportunities ignored since Brown v. Board of Education: Youth development and the myth of a color-blind society. *Educational Researcher, 37,* 253–266.

Thornton, M.C., Chatters, L.M., Taylor, R.J., & Allen, W. (1990). Sociodemographic and environmental correlates of racial socialization by Black parents. *Child Development, 61,* 401–409.

Yoshikawa, H. (2011). Immigrants raising citizens: Undocumented parents and their young children. New York: Russell Sage Foundation.

US Census Bureau (2010). Population Statistics.

Deborah J. Johnson, PhD
Department of Human Development and Family Studies, 103 HE BLDG
Michigan State University
East Lansing, MI 48824 (USA)
Tel. +1 517 432 9115
E-Mail john1442@hdfs.msu.edu

Dr. Deborah J. Johnson (PhD 1988, Northwestern University) is Professor of Human Development and Family Studies at Michigan State University. Her research focuses on the racialized and culturally-related parenting and development of African American and other children, both domestically and globally. In particular, she has been interested in how parental messages and context influence the racial coping responses of children. She has also been interested in the global contexts of these aspects of development among vulnerable children in Africa and Australia. Conceptual and theoretical scholarship has emphasized disentangling race, culture, and poverty and furthering ethnic/racial socialization paradigms. Her published work has appeared in books, monographs, articles and chapters.

Paper

Slaughter-Defoe DT (ed): Racial Stereotyping and Child Development.
Contrib Hum Dev. Basel, Karger, 2012, vol 25, pp 28–46

Media Socialization, Black Media Images and Black Adolescent Identity

Valerie N. Adams[a] · Howard C. Stevenson, Jr.[b]

[a]Cornell University, Ithaca, N.Y., and [b]University of Pennsylvania, Pa., USA

Abstract

Media exposure, particularly for children and youth, has been demonstrated to be a powerful tool used to brand images, and, in the case of public health campaigns, to impart knowledge and influence behavioral change. Importantly, this generation of youth is living in a more culturally diverse society then prior generations and has access to multiple media platforms that feature Black people. Unfortunately, the selection of Blacks – defined as any person of African descent – presented in mainstream media is often limited to a discrete group of Black celebrities or stereotypical images. How Black youth interpret negative stereotype images of Black people promulgated in the media has not adequately been explored. The research presented in this chapter references American media that feature Black/African American actors and actresses. The study presented investigated the relationships among exposure to negative stereotype Black media images, racial identity, racial socialization, body image and self-esteem for 14- to 21-year-old Black youth. This chapter applies the concepts of racial identity and racial/ethnic socialization (R/ES) [Bentley, Adams & Stevenson, 2009; Stevenson, 2011] to the study results that suggest: (a) the youth perceive that persistent negative messages about Black people still exist, and (b) these messages continue to influence youth perspectives and have the potential to influence identity development processes.

Copyright © 2012 S. Karger AG, Basel

Media exposure, for children [Calvert, 2008] and youth [Bush, Smith & Martin, 1999], has been demonstrated to be a powerful tool used to brand images, and, in the case of public health campaigns, to impart knowledge and influence behavioral change [Evans, 2008; Grier & Bryant, 2005; Walsh, Rudd, Moeykens & Moloney, 1993]. Today's youth are living in a more culturally diverse society then prior generations and have access to multiple media platforms that feature Black people. Unfortunately, the selection of Black images – defined as any person of African descent – presented in mainstream media is often limited to a discrete group of Black celebrities or stereotypes [Gorham, 1999; Jackson, 2006; Ramasubramanian, 2007].

Characters who embody negative stereotypes about Black people have dominated the U.S. media and entertainment industry throughout history [Allen & Bielby, 1977; Allen & Thornton, 1992; Bogle, 2001a, b; Jackson, 2006]. Bogle's [Bogle, 1973, 2001b] *Toms, Coons, Mulattoes, Mammies & Bucks: An Interpretive History of Blacks in American Films* is an exhaustive chronicle of Black characters spanning eight decades. Early film and television shows featured White actors in blackface whose character portrayals were exaggerated or distorted representations of Black people as uncivilized, illiterate, and/or unintelligent, with little sense of direction and in need of guidance; other characterizations depicted Blacks as subservient hired help whose primary desire was to please their White employers [Bogle, 1973; Jackson, 2006]. Jackson [2006] notes:

> Over the course of 150 years from 1769 to about 1927, minstrelsy would become an institution, revered by Whites for its dehumanizing yet somehow entertaining characterization of Blacks as darkies and Whites as ordinary, normal, and cultured ladies and gentlemen . . . indicative of both their attitudes about Blacks and their own self-perceptions[1] (p. 21).

Besides the minstrel-inspired 'coons' and 'mammies,' additional stereotypical characterizations became staple images of Black females ('tragic mulatto'; 'sapphire'; 'jezebel') and males ('Buck'; 'Uncle Tom'[2]) [Bogle, 1973, 1980, 2001a, 2001b; Jackson, 2006].

Both Bogle [1973] and Jackson [2006] carefully describe the precarious position of Black actors and actresses[3] who starred in these roles during earlier decades when the possibility of fair and equitable treatment for Black Americans was extremely limited and influenced by societal norms. In spite of social advances, there remains within the TV and film industry a practice of presenting negative stereotype images of Black people scripted from early characters[4] predicated on social assumptions about the racial inferiority of Blacks [Allen & Thornton, 1992; Bogle, 2001a, b; Gorham, 1999; Jackson, 2006].

While consensus has grown about the prevalence of negative Black media images, measuring the influence of these images on Black youth self-perceptions and the influence of youth rejection or endorsement of these images on their well-being and identity is a new and understudied phenomenon.

In the United States, a small number of studies show that Black adults find a relationship between racism and media imagery; researchers found Black adults to be critical of TV images they perceived to represent negative stereotype messages about Black people, and as a result of these images, they were mistrustful of TV as a credible source of information about Black life [Allen & Bielby, 1977; Allen & Thornton, 1992; Davis & Gandy, 1999]. While fewer studies have found this relationship for youth, researchers have begun to question how racial identity or socialization influence media interpretation, media preferences and the body images of Black youth [Gordon, 2008; O'Connor, Brooks-Gunn & Graber, 2000; Ward, 2004]. Research in this chapter focuses on how Black youth interpret negative stereotype media images of Black/African American actors and actresses. Specifically, the study reported in this chapter investigated the relationships between exposure to negative stereotype Black media images[5], racial identity, racial socialization, body image and self-esteem for 14- to 21-year-old Black youth. Using the theoretical lens of racial identity and racial/ethnic socialization (R/ES) [Bentley, Adams & Stevenson, 2009; Stevenson, 2011; Stevenson & Arrington, 2009], the authors suggest that: (a) youth perceive that persistent negative messages about Black people still exist, and (b) these messages continue to influence youth perspectives and identity development processes.

---

[1] See Jackson [2006], pp. 20–24, for a detailed discussion of this phenomenon.
[2] Bogle [2001b] discusses the introduction of the 'sidekick' as a contemporary negatively stereotyped characterization of Blacks.
[3] Black actors and actresses in earlier decades of TV and film were aware of the negative portrayals they embodied on screen. Cognizant of the limited opportunities for Black actors and actresses and of the importance of Blacks being seen on TV and in movies, they played the characters. Some would attempt to infuse the characters with a degree of dignity or resilience. Off stage, many were involved in Civil Rights initiatives, supported equal opportunities for Black Americans, and invested in community-level programming for Blacks [Bogle, 1973].
[4] Jackson [2006] and Bogle [2001a, b] detail other characterizations of Blacks that are premised on the same assumptions that underlie the stock negative profiles.

[5] Positive stereotype media images of Black people also exist [Allen & Thornton, 1992; Berry, 1998]. Both negative and positive stereotype media messages that occur in print and TV media were examined in this study.

Media Socialization

Media socialization lays the foundation for how youth come to acquire static or stereotypic self- and other representations. There appears to be no consensus on a definition for media socialization even though it is consistently referenced in research. Dennis McQuail defines media socialization as the process of teaching norms and values by way of symbolic reward and punishment for different kinds of behavior as represented in the media; or a learning process whereby people learn how to behave in certain situations and the expectations which coincide with a given role or status in society [McQuail, 2005]. Heide [1995] defines media socialization as 'the manner in which we establish a relationship to social reality through media representation'. It has also been defined as the internalization of attentional cues via a 'thorough initiation into the terrain of television's forms and conventions'. Attentional cues are described as formal features of active viewing that guide an individual's cognitive processing [Biocca, 1988].

Using the aforementioned definitions, we define media socialization as the exposure to mass communication (television, radio, internet, newspapers) messages, which teach people socially accepted behaviors that have: (a) a direct influence on cognitive ability and behavioral functioning, and (b) a mediating or facilitative indirect influence on learning.

Media Socialization Paradigms

There are two established paradigms of media socialization. The traditional paradigm is the basis for many of the early studies with media, children, and youth and is concerned with how media[6] is used and its effects on cognitive development and behavior [Arnett, Larson & Offer, 1995; Wartella, O'Keefe & Scantlin, 2000]. The Bobo doll study is an example of the type of studies that are concerned with the effect of exposure on behavior [Bandura, Ross & Ross, 1963; Plomin, Foch & Rowe, 1981]. The second paradigm considers how different kinds of media can be used to stimulate cognitive growth [Wartella, O'Keefe & Scantlin, 2000]. This paradigm is not as concerned with establishing how cognitive capabilities are used to interpret media; rather it is helpful for understanding how children learn from different mediums. Studies within this paradigm are concerned with how media products designed to stimulate the cognitive abilities of children can enhance and/or facilitate learning, i.e., *Sesame Street* and video game studies [Browne Graves, 1982].

Recent research with adolescents has identified a third paradigm in which media acts as an influential socializing agent because of increased exposure [Berry, 1998]. This newer paradigm is influenced by the number of hours adolescents are exposed to media via *multitasking* – the practice of using multiple technologies at once [Strasburger, Wilson & Jordan, 2009]. TV remains the largest medium of exposure by far, but cell phone, computer, radio, and video games are elements of consideration for multitasking [Brown & Marin, 2009; Roberts & Foehr, 2008] and require cognitive skills[7] to manage several of these mediums simultaneously.

The present generation of youth is exposed to media images at least 100 times more than youth in prior generations [Roberts & Foehr, 2008]. Studies of how media influence the cognitive functioning of children and youth show that White and Black youth have different television viewing habits. African-American children spend a significantly higher number of hours viewing TV than White youth. Not only do African American youth have the highest level of TV consumption compared to their peers [Bickham et al., 2003;

---

[6] Classic studies examined exposure to television. Some researchers continue to employ the same definition with contemporary studies of TV, video games, and other mediums.

[7] The increase in access to technologically based media platforms has resulted in a body of research that examines how and whether multi-tasking impacts cognitive functioning.

Blosser, 1988; Roberts & Foehr, 2008; Tynes & Ward, 2009; Wartella et al., 2000], but also entertainment is the primary reason for this consumption [Berry, 1998; Bickham et al., 2003; Gordon, 2008; Lee & Browne, 1981; Ward, 2004; Ward, Day & Epstein, 2006]. In 1988, Blosser worked with a sample of 349 Black, White, Puerto Rican, and Mexican children ages 5–15 to examine differences in quantity of use, frequency of use, access to media, and media usage habits. The study found Black youth watch more TV during the school day, after school, and during the evening than White and Hispanic youth [Blosser, 1988]. Roberts' census of children's and youth's media habits found Black youth dedicated 48% of their media diet to TV viewing, compared to White youth, whose viewing equaled 38% [Roberts, 2000]. Both Blosser [1988] and Roberts [2000] found Black youth reported higher levels of playing video games and going to movies than White youth.

Body image and sexuality are powerful factors in adolescent personal and racial identity development. Media studies with African-American youth provide a framework for how media exposure influences body image ideals [O'Connor et al., 2000; Parker, 1999], self-esteem [O'Connor et al., 2000], and sexuality [Arnett et al., 1995; Escobar-Chaves & Anderson, 2008; Ward, Day et al., 2006]. In spite of the increase in media studies that focus on Black youth, studies that examine the relationship of racial identity to how to how Black youth interpret and respond to media images of Black people remain scarce.

Theories of Media-Generated Racial/Ethnic Socialization

Cultivation Theory. Two theories serve as a framework for this research: Cultivation Theory [Gerbner & Gross, 1976] and Phenomenological Variant of Ecological Systems Theory (PVEST) [Spencer, 1995]. Gerbner's cultivation theory [1976] is premised upon the assumption that television viewing is the primary source of storytelling in American society. This theory suggests that higher rates of TV exposures are associated with internalizing the stories (images) as representative of reality. High-volume viewers exposed to repeated messages are theorized to adapt a 'mean world view' – a view of the world as worse than it actually is, and a resulting mistrust of people around them [Gerbner, 1998; Gerbner & Gross, 1976]. Cultivation theory has proven consistently useful for confirming associations between level of TV exposure and real-life perceptions [Gerbner, 1998]. Applying cultivation theory to the TV-viewing habits of Black youth, who have the highest number of viewing hours and a preference for Black TV shows [Berry, 1998; Watkins, 2000], suggests that youth will accept Black character portrayals and media images as valid models of acceptable and expected behaviors for Black people. Still, cultivation theory doesn't address the nuances of Black culture, the history of racial oppression, or the ongoing use of racial stereotyping in contemporary Black life, social and economic mobility and stagnation.

Phenomenological Variant of Ecological Systems Theory. An integrated perspective on how macro- and systemic racial insults influence Black cultural and individual functioning and identity can be found in the Phenomenological Variant of Ecological Systems Theory (PVEST). PVEST allows for contextual analysis of behavior by assessing vulnerability level, net stress, reactive coping strategies, emergent identities, and life stage outcomes[8] relative to the experiences of African American youth. In determining vulnerability level – protective factors (those which help to shield youth from stressors) and risk contributors (those things which heighten vulnerability and stress reaction), racial attitudes and behaviors can be incorporated into the analysis of the experiences of

---

[8] Vulnerability level, net stress, reactive coping strategies, emergent identities, and life stage outcomes are the five elements of PVEST. See Spencer [2006] for detailed definitions of all of the elements.

African American youth [Spencer, 1995, 2006]. Net stress, the second component of PVEST, permits examination of how risks (such as racism) that youth confront are counteracted by available supports (i.e., family structure, neighborhood composition, or friends); the quality and quantity of supports available to youth influence their reactive coping strategies – which may be adaptive or maladaptive. African-American youth are frequently tasked with developing healthy, positive emergent identities[9] as part of adolescence by navigating around conflicting messages received from media, family, friends, and teachers, along with interpreting racialized experiences and developing necessary coping strategies [Spencer, 1995; Spencer, Dupree, Swanson & Cunningham, 1996]. Vulnerability level, net stress, and reactive coping strategies are the first three elements of PVEST and were used to frame the study presented in this chapter.

The authors of this chapter assume that this generation's increased exposure to the manipulated media imagery and the global distribution of *Blackness* beyond television are considered vulnerability level risks, and that exposure to Black images in the media will correlate with racial socialization, racial identity, body image, and self-esteem processes (scores). Within the context of net stress engagement, racial/ethnic socialization, and self-esteem may be considered supports or challenges. High scores for each of the listed variables are expected to represent net stress supports that can serve as buffers against the influence of exposure to negative Black media images. Racial/ethnic socialization (R/ES) is theorized as a lens through which an individual's perceptions of self and, racial/ethnic group identity and coping options are appraised [Stevenson, 2011]. Despite the influence of macro-systemic racial factors in PVEST and cultivation theories there is less

explanation on the more proximal mechanisms that youth use to accept or reject negative images of Blacks through media. R/ES research attempts to address this gap by illuminating the multiple developmental influences on youth racial identity in more proximal, dyadic relational contexts.

Racial/Ethnic Socialization (R/ES). As parents and family members are primary socializing agents for youth, they model for youth how to consider, manage, resolve racial and ethnic dynamics through verbal and nonverbal interactions and communications. This interaction process between family and youth has been called racial/ethnic socialization (R/ES). Many Black parents practice racial/ethnic socialization in order to help youth to buffer and transcend negative messages and experiences they may encounter about being Black [Barr & Neville, 2008; Bentley et al., 2009; Hughes et al., 2006; Stevenson & Arrington, 2009]. However, because of increasing levels of exposure, media, not just family, is also a socializing agent, providing youth with messages about societal norms and modeling expected behaviors [Arnett, 1995; Berry, 2000; Stroman, 1991].

Given the historical legacy of Black media representations, high levels of media viewing, and the importance of identity development during adolescence, we will explore what relationships exist among exposure to Black media stereotypes, racial socialization, and the racial identity of Black adolescents. Admittedly, media interpretations and viewing preferences are influenced by a variety of factors such as family composition, income, gender, age, and the education level of parents [Arnett, 1995; Wartella et al., 2000].

Measuring Youth Perceptions of Media-Generated Racial/Ethnic Socialization

A key problem in the literature presented is the lack of measurement on Black media messages, beliefs, and frequency of use. Currently, there is no standardized measure for identifying Black media message stereotypes. Studies that identify

---

[9] Within the PVEST framework emergent identities may be positive or negative. The access youth have to protective factors and supports influence their coping behaviors, which ultimately shapes their emergent identities.

and/or investigate media stereotypes ask for respondents' impressions of media images by employing a strategy of referencing videos, TV shows, and/or characters [Allen & Bielby, 1979; Allen & Thornton, 1992; Fujioka, 2005; Gordon, 2008; Ward, 2004; Ward, Hansbrough & Walker, 2005] that are or were current during the time the study was conducted. News-media-oriented studies use current event stories or mainstream versus Black media outlets [Vercellotti & Brewer, 2006] as a reference for investigating stereotype messages about Black people. Studies of female stereotype images employ a content analysis strategy framed by common negative portrayals of Black females in the media [Balaji, 2008, 2009; Woodard & Mastin, 2005]. In fact, content analysis is a common methodology for analyzing media content. However, this strategy does not ask participants to identify the stereotypes. Rather, researchers frame the analysis using common stereotypical constructs that are applied to Black media content.

There are also studies with youth that ask participants how they relate to specific characters and/or about viewing preferences: mainstream TV shows or Black-oriented TV shows [Gordon, 2008; Ward, 2004; Ward, Day et al., 2006; Ward et al., 2005]. These studies sometimes include still images, but commonly reference TV shows and characters without asking participants to identify the implicit message(s) associated with the characters or TV shows being referenced. Creating a measure that focuses on the respondents' ability to identify the messages associated with media images will help researchers to further study and measure how media socialization operates within the developmental experiences of Black adolescents.

Certainly the influence of sociohistoric factors on the story lines and characters that appear on TV shows is a critique of creating an instrument that uses still images to analyze media stereotypes. We assume the implicit argument against creating the instrument is that characters and TV shows will lose their context and relevance over time because the story lines were written to reflect the current events and social norms during the show's original airing. This critique suggests characters featured on current/real-time TV shows may not retain their meaning(s) with future generations introduced to the characters or images during a different time period. However, analyses demonstrate the persistence of negative Black media content in spite of industry advances and the introduction of positive Black media images [Bogle, 2001a, b; Coltrane & Messineo, 2000; Jackson, 2006; Nama, 2003; Watkins, 2000; Woodard & Mastin, 2005]. Advanced technology preserves discontinued shows for viewing by current and future generations. Up-to-date shows cloak traditional stereotypes in contemporary characters by using modern colloquial language, clothing, gadgets, and in some case surrounding Black characters with multicultural casts. As such, the media racial socialization of negative Black stereotypes persists across generations since older shows are retained, old stereotypical characters are not modified despite contemporary contexts and frames, and no counter socialization strategies are presented in contemporary shows to debate the negative portrayals of these stereotypes.

The Black Media Message Questionnaire: A Measure of Black Media Stereotypes

The Black Media Message Questionnaire (BMMQ) was created for use with Black adolescents to determine if they would be able to identify stereotype messages associated with images of Black people on TV and in print magazines; assess their belief of media messages identified, and to estimate the frequency of exposure to the message selected when watching TV and/or reading magazines [Adams & Stevenson, 2011].

The support for the creation of a measure of how youth experience the negative imaging of Black characters include the following assumptions: (1) print and television media present stereotypes of Black people, often negative, and (2) these images inform and influence adolescent perspectives about Black people that some accept as real-life representations.

Research Question

Important research questions raised in this chapter examine the relationships among exposure to media images of Black people, racial identity, and racial socialization for Black adolescents and their endorsement of the negative messages associated with these images. Secondary research questions explore how racial/ethnic socialization and Black identity are associated with self-esteem, and body image.

Method

Given the evidence provided by prior research and the importance of the adolescent identity process, using the BMMQ, we conducted a study to explore relationships between media exposure and the adolescent identity process of Black youth. This study sought to determine whether Black adolescents are able to identify Black racial stereotypes in the media; to determine if Black youth endorse Black media stereotypes, how often they are exposed to these stereotypes, and whether their exposure and endorsement of Black media stereotypes is related to racial socialization, racial identity, body image, or self-esteem scores. Although there were multiple questions addressed in this study, the results presented in this chapter will only focus on the relationships we believe are most important to consider when thinking about media socialization and the development processes Black adolescents experience.

Research Sample

A group of 113 Black adolescents ages 14- to 21-year-old were recruited to participate in this study because these groups represent two different stages of adolescence where shifts in self-image, peer groups, and aspirations are relevant and evolving as adult identities began to emerge. Beauty, attractiveness, personal image, and identity are relevant to both age groups. Among middle adolescents the importance of belonging, academic achievement, peer groups, and social contexts are of major concern. Late-stage adolescents have similar concerns but their decisions and attention are aligned with career choices. Their tasks and affiliations, both professional and personal, are chosen dependent on these near-future aspirations.

This study posed questions about age, mother's and father's educational level, income, and gender to obtain basic

descriptive information about the sample. Multi-layered racial background information allowed data to be gathered about respondent's biracial, multiracial, and Black Diasporic (African, Caribbean, Hispanic) backgrounds.

Of the 113 respondents, 44% were 14- to 17-year-old and 56% were 18 to 21 years old. Sixty-four percent of the respondents identified as Black/African American, 9% identified as Black Caribbean, 8% identified as Multiracial, 5% identified as White, 4% identified as Black African, 4% identified as Other. Fifty-six percent were between the ages of 18 and 21 with a mean age of 18. Sixty-four percent of respondents were female, 36% were male, with 49% identifying as high school students, 46% as college students, 4% as middle school students and 2%[10] as other – a recent college graduate and trade school student. Study participants reported a mean GPA of 3.00 to 3.24, with students attending Catholic, charter, public and private high schools or colleges. In line with the findings of existing research, TV viewing was high: 41% indicated 4 to 6 hours of TV watching per week. Twenty-seven percent indicated 7 or more hours of TV viewing per week.

Measures

Black Media Messages Questionnaire. The BMMQ consists of 4 subscales. Twenty image items are repeatedly used for each of the 4 subscales; each item has a media image followed by four statements [Adams, 2009]. The first subscale is entitled *Black Media Message (BMMS)* For this scale youth *are asked to select the statement you believe best represents the message presented by this image.* This scale is designed for participants to identify the messages believed to be represented by the media image. The statements for each item reflect both gender and body image themes and views that are either positive or negative. After selecting one of the messages associated with the image, the second subscale Black Media Message Belief Subscale (BMMB) of the BMMQ instructed youth to indicate how much they agreed with the message they had selected for the BMMS. The *Black Media Message Belief* scale is reflected in the question *How much do you agree with this message?*

The third subscale is entitled Black Media Message TV Frequency (BMMTV-Freq) and is reflected in the question *When viewing TV (cable, dish TV, movies, sitcoms, dramas) how often do you see images that present this message?* Lastly, for the fourth subscale, participants were asked about frequency of viewing the selected message in magazines. This subscale is entitled *Black Media Message Magazine Frequency* (BMMMag-Freq) and is reflected in the question *When flipping through magazines how often do you see images that present this message?* The response options for these two scales were *never, hardly ever (1–2), lots of times (4–6),* and *all of the time (7 or more*

---

[10] Percentages were rounded up to whole numbers.

times). The BMMTV-Freq and the BMMMag-Freq scales were designed to measure the frequency of exposure to Black media messages on TV and in magazines[11]. Each of the BMMQ scales has a positive (P) and a negative (N) factor.

Multidimensional Inventory of Black Identity-Teen (Mibi-T). The MIBI-T is a measure of the extent to which race is relevant to the self-concept at a particular point in time or in a particular situation [Scottham, Sellers & Nguyên, 2008]. It consists of four aspects of racial identity: how a person defines themselves in terms of race (Centrality); how a person evaluates their racial group (regard – assessed in terms of both Public and Private Regard); and how they think members of the racial group act (ideology – Humanist, Oppressed minority, Nationalist, and Assimilationist). The Centrality, Public and Private Regard scales are the primary aspects used for the analyses in this study.

Youth were instructed to choose the response that represented their agreement on a 5-point Likert scale ranging from 1 *(really disagree)* to 5 *(really agree)* with statements representative of each scale. For example, 'I have a strong sense of belonging to other Black people' is from the Centrality scale; 'Most people think that Blacks are as smart as people of other races' is an example from the Public Regard scale; 'I am happy that I am Black' is an example from the Private Regard scale. Exploratory zero order correlations were conducted with each of the factors from the BMMQ scales and the two racial identity scales.

Cultural and Racial Experiences of Socialization (CARES). The CARES survey is a 53-item scale that measures the acquisition of racial socialization messages; it gauges the frequency (exposure), endorsement (internalization), and source of messages [Bentley & Stevenson, 2011]. The CARES has 6 subscales: Alertness to Racism; Bi-Cultural Coping; Racial Legacy Knowledge; Cultural Pride; Internalized Racialism; Stereotyping. The present study utilizes only the CARES Exposure and Endorsement subscale scores. For the exposure subscale, after reading each message, participants are asked about the frequency of receiving the message *(not at all, sometimes, or all of the time)*, and the endorsement scale asks to what extent they agree with the message *(strongly disagree, disagree, agree, or strongly agree)*.

Sociocultural Attitudes Towards Appearance Scale-3 (SATAQ-3). Body image was measured using the SATAQ-3, which is a 30-item, 4-factor self-report measure of body image [Thompson, Patricia, Roehrig, Guarda & Heinberg, 2004]. Information, Pressures, Internalization General, and Internalization Athlete are the four factors for this scale. The Information subscale assesses the perceived

importance of media for obtaining information about 'being attractive'. The Information subscale is referred to as Attraction Ideal. The Pressures subscale assesses feeling pressured by media to strive for cultural ideals of physical appearance. The Internalization-General subscale assesses endorsement and acceptance of media messages that present unrealistic ideal images. Internalization-General is referred to as Unrealistic Ideal. The Internalization-Athletic scale assesses endorsement and acceptance of an athletic body ideal. It is referred to as Ideal Athletic Body.

The Rosenberg Self-Esteem (RSE) scale was used to measure self-esteem. This is a 10-item self-report measure with a total possible score of 30 [Rosenberg, 1989]. In the next section, we present a selection of results that align with our interest in learning about relationships among media socialization, racial identity, racial socialization, self-esteem and body image.

Results

Relationships of Demographic Variables to BMMQ Factors. Exploratory zero order correlations were conducted with all BMMQ variables. The demographic variables examined were *youth's race, father's race, mother's race, father's education, mother's education, parents' marital status, family income, experience with racist acts, experience of racist acts against a family member, family talks about racism, expected level of educational attainment, TV viewing hours, magazine reading hours, varsity sport participation, extracurricular activity participation, age, developmental age,* and *gender*.

BMMB Correlations. The BMMB factors were examined first. The P-BMMB factor was only found to have a significant relationship with age ($r = 0.21$, $p < 0.05$). There were 3 significant inverse correlations for the N-BMMB factor: family income ($r = -0.22$, $p < 0.05$), expected level of education attainment ($r = -0.21$, $p < 0.05$), and extracurricular activity participation ($r = -0.29$, $p < 0.01$). Youth with higher family income, educational attainment and more participation in extracurricular activities were less likely to endorse negative stereotype messages.

BMMTV-Freq Correlations. There was one significant correlation for P-BMMTV-Freq: age

---

[11] See Adams and Stevenson [2011] for a detailed description of the BMMQ measure.

(r = –0.22, p < 0.05); older youth report lower frequencies of witnessing positive Black stereotype media messages on TV. N-BMMTV-Freq was significantly correlated with 2 variables: mother's education (r = 0.22, p < 0.05), and age (r = 0.41, p < 0.01). The higher the education level of the student's mother and age of the student, the more students reported frequently witnessing negative Black stereotype television messages.

BMMMag-Freq Correlations. Only age (r = 0.32, p < 0.01), significantly correlated with N-BMMMag-Freq; older youth scored higher in witnessing negative Black media messages in magazines. There were no significant correlations with P-BMMag-Freq.

Correlation Analysis of Racial Identity to BMMQ. This analysis was conducted to address the following hypotheses: racial identity, Regard, and Centrality will have a significant relationship with Black media message belief. Three factors from the MIBI-T were used for this analysis. Private Regard was the only positive and statistically significant factor (r = 0.29, p < 0.01) for P-BMMB. Youth with higher Private Regard scores were more likely to assert that the positive statement attached to the Black media image was the correct message. Private Regard scores had an inverse relationship and were significantly correlated (r = –0.22, p < 0.05) with N-BMMB. This was an expected finding.

It was also expected that youth with high private regard scores and high centrality scores would not agree that the negative statement accurately represented the Black media image and thus score lower on this subscale. Significant relationships for Private Regard partially supported the hypothesis that racial identity would have a significant relationship with the BMMB factors.

BMMTV-Freq Correlations. This analysis was conducted to test the hypothesis that racial identity will have a significant relationship with the frequency of the types of Black media messages identified on TV. There were no significant correlations for P-BMMTV-Freq. N-BMMTV-Freq scores were inversely and significantly (r = –0.21, p < 0.05) correlated with Public Regard scores. The results of this analysis partially support the tested hypothesis: Youth with high Public Regard scores reported that the negative stereotype images and messages did not frequently appear on television.

BMMMAG-Freq Correlations. This analysis was conducted to test the hypothesis that racial identity would have a significant relationship with frequency of Black media messages in magazines. None of the racial identity variables were significantly correlated with P-BMMMag-Freq or N-BMMMag-Freq scores. In general, magazine reading was low for this sample, which could explain the lack of significant findings.

It was expected that there would be a significant relationship between Centrality and BMMQ scores for each scale. This hypothesis was not supported – none of the BMMQ factors were significantly correlated with Centrality. An examination of TV viewing and magazine reading showed higher Centrality scores were significantly (r = –0.19, p < 0.05) and inversely correlated with watching TV and inversely correlated (r = –0.08, p < 0.05) with reading magazines. Youth with higher Centrality score reported watching fewer hours of TV and spending fewer hours reading magazines.

Correlation Analysis of Racial Socialization Experience
To address the hypothesis that youth high in racial socialization will also score high on the factors of the Black media message measure, exploratory zero order correlations were conducted between the factors of the BMMQ and CARES scales. The CARES consists of three measures: *CARES Frequency* asks youth *Have your parents/ relatives, friends/peers, teachers/professors, other adults, or the media said to you any of the following statements throughout your lifetime? How*

often? CARES Agreement asks youth *How much do you agree?* with the statements; *CARES Source* asks *Where did you hear this?* This research study was designed to assess exposure to racial socialization experience; because of this the five factors for CARES Frequency were tabulated for each youth and were used in the remaining analyses.

There are five CARES factors that represent the types of racial socialization messages that youth report receiving. The Racial/Ethnic (R/E) Affirmation factor is composed of items that represent messages that positively uphold and support the experiences of Black people. These messages often include a reference to historical/ cultural experiences, i.e., 'To be Black is to be connected to a history that goes back to African royalty'. The R/E Protection factor is composed of items that represent statements that can help youth guard against racially stressful encounters, i.e., 'You should speak up when someone says something that is racist'. The R/E Stereotype factor includes items about messages that express negative perspectives (internalized racism) about Black people, i.e., 'Some Black people are just born with good hair'. The R/E Regard for Whiteness factors includes messages about encounters and preferences for Whiteness, i.e., 'Black children will learn more if they go to a mostly white school'. The R/E Competence Resolution factor includes statements about how youth use particular coping strategies in dealing with differential treatment because they are Black, i.e., 'Fitting into school or work means swallowing your anger when you see racism'.

Black Media Message Belief (BMMB) Correlations. Correlations with the BMMB factors were examined first to address the hypothesis that Black Media Message Belief (BMMB) scores would have a significant relationship with racial socialization experience (CARES scores). Surprisingly, there were no significant correlations with any of the CARES factors for N-BMMB, although Regard for Whiteness appeared to be approaching significance ($r = -0.18$, $p < 0.06$) for N-

BMMB. There were significant correlations with P-BMMB for Protection ($r = 0.26$, $p < 0.01$) and Affirmation, ($r = 0.31$, $p < 0.01$). It seems youth with higher Protection and Affirmation scores were more likely to believe positive media messages about Black people.

The hypothesis for this analysis predicted there would be significant relationships between the BMMB and CARES variables. The results partially support this hypothesis. It was expected there would be a significant relationship between N-BMMB scores and the CARES Stereotype and Regard for Whiteness factors. These two factors did begin to approach significance; therefore it is possible a larger sample size would result in significance for individual CARES factors.

Black Media Message TV Frequency (BMMTV-Freq) Correlations. Correlations between the BMMTV-Freq factors and the CARES factors were examined. There were no significant correlations for P-BMMTV-Freq, although Affirmation appeared to be approaching significance. N-BMMTV-Freq was significantly correlated with five factors: Protection ($r = 0.33$, $p < 0.01$), Stereotype ($r = 0.34$, $p < 0.01$), Regard for Whiteness ($r = 0.32$, $p < 0.01$), and Competence ($r = 0.21$, $p < 0.05$). Youth with high scores for these factors were more likely to report seeing more negative stereotype messages on television.

The hypotheses for this analysis predicted there would be significant relationships between the BMMTV-frequency and CARES variables. The results of the correlation analysis partially supported this hypothesis. Youth with higher scores on these variables were more likely to identify negative messages about Black people when watching TV. The non-significant relationship between racial socialization and P-BMMTV-Freq may be appropriate. It follows that youth with higher racial socialization scores would be likely to report negative media messages, which are prevalent, and unlikely to identify positive messages when watching TV because they are almost non-existent.

Black Media Message Magazine Frequency (BMMMag-Freq) Correlations. A third set of correlations was performed to test the hypothesis that frequency of Black messages in magazines (BMMMag-Freq scores) would have a significant relationship with racial socialization experience (CARES scores). One variable, Affirmation (r = 0.21, p < 0.05), was significantly correlated with P-BMMMag-Freq. N-BMMMag-Freq was significantly correlated with three factors; Protection (r = 0.26, p < 0.01) Regard for Whiteness, (r = 0.26, p < 0.01) and Stereotype (r = 0.22, p < 0.05).

This hypothesis also predicted there would be significant relationships between the BMMMag-Freq and CARES variables. There was one variable significantly correlated with P-BMMMag-Freq and three significantly correlated with N-BMMMag-Freq. The results of these analyses suggest youth with high levels of racial socialization significantly report greater frequency of negative media messages about Black people in magazines.

Correlation Analysis of Self-Esteem to BMMQ Factors
Exploratory zero order correlations were conducted between the BMMQ factor scores and RSE self-esteem scores to address the hypotheses that there would be a relationship between these variables. There were no statistically significant relationships between self-esteem scores and any of the BMMQ factors. Our hypothesis was not supported. However, esteem scores were inversely related to five of the factors. The P-BMMB factor was the only factor positively correlated with self-esteem; youth with higher self-esteem scores were more likely to believe positive stereotype messages about Black people.

Correlation Analysis of Body Image
Exploratory zero order correlations were conducted between the BMMQ factor scores and body image (SATAQ-3) scores to address the hypotheses that there would be a relationship between these

variables. There were no statistically significant relationships with body image. Only P-BMMB was positively correlated with all four of the body image factors. P-BMMTV-Freq, N-BMMTV-Freq, and N-BMMB were all negatively correlated with the Attraction Ideal, Pressures, Unrealistic Ideal, and Ideal Athletic Body factors. P-BMMMag-Freq and N-BMMMag-Freq were negatively correlated with Attraction Ideal, Unrealistic Ideal, and Ideal Athletic Body. The hypothesis for this analysis was not supported, but the direction of the relationships between SATAQ-3 and BMMQ scores suggests lower body image scores are associated with media exposure.

Discussion

Empirical Findings
The main research question for this study was, 'What are the relationships among degree of exposure to images of Blacks in the media, racial/ethnic socialization, and racial identity for 14- to 21-year-old Black adolescents?' This study also sought to investigate what relationships exist among exposure to images of Blacks in the media and: (a) body image, and (b) self-esteem scores of Black adolescents. To address these questions, this study focused on TV and print media images because TV remains the highest-ranking medium of use for African-American youth and because African-American households often subscribe to magazines targeting Black audiences. These magazines feature stories about Black life and include advertisements that use predominantly Black models, actors or actresses.

This study applied the concepts of racial identity and racial/ethnic socialization (R/ES) to the research on exposure to Black media images to assess how Black young people interpret associated messages. Black characters that reflect negative stereotype images of Black people constantly appear on prime-time television and shows targeted toward Black audiences. Black youth who are high viewers of media are exposed to a high volume of images that often project negative stereotype messages about Black people.

The concern that Black American youth may accept negative stereotype TV images of Black people as valid, resulting in a negative impact on identity and self-esteem, was the basis of this research study. Racial socialization studies with youth have traditionally focused on message transfer between people, not between media and people. Existing studies fall short of exploring relationships that may exist between Black racial identity and R/E socialization with exposure to Black media images for Black adolescent youth. Disappointingly, research that examines racial identity and R/E socialization as influencing media exposure, body image, and self-esteem are also scant.

For Blacks, racism is a significant cultural factor influencing identity exploration. The racial/ethnic socialization youth experience serves as the reference for how youth interpret messages about Black people and helps them to identify messages as positive or negative. Many prime-time TV shows do not include Black characters [Jefferson, 1970; Nama, 2003; Watkins, 2000]. Thus, Black children, youth, and adults watch Black-oriented half-hour sitcoms that tend to be racially segregated, but feature an all-Black or majority Black cast [Jefferson, 1970; Watkins, 2000]. Although the representations of Black TV images evolve to reflect sociohistoric moments in time, negative stereotypes persist [Nama, 2003].

In this study we expected interpretation and endorsement of Black media images to be mediated by racial socialization and self-esteem. Further, we expected youth racial identity and body image to be positively correlated with media exposure and racial socialization scores. In addition, we predicted that youth with high racial socialization scores would have high racial identity, body image, and self-esteem scores. We assumed that one's gender, age, and personal experience of racist acts were three demographic variables that would be important in this research. With

regard to gender, there were significant differences in identifying media messages as positive or negative for females versus males. Younger youth identified more positive media images than older youth. This could be a reflection of TV viewing habits; younger youth's media diet may be inclusive of TV shows targeting preteens and younger adolescents. These shows make more attempts to appeal to the cognitive processes of children and youth. Research supports the idea that Black youth watch TV for entertainment [Berry, 1998; Browne Graves, 1982; Watkins, 2000]; it could also be that since younger youth have less exposure to negative racial experiences than older youth they are less sensitive to these messages when presented in media.

Males were less likely to identify negative media stereotypes, but more likely to endorse them than females. Gendered media stereotypes of Black women are very often sexualized [Balaji, 2008]. Puberty and the early maturation of Black girls are probable influences on how females perceive Black media images, particularly those associated with body image. The gender socialization experience and messages that men receive about women are likely to influence their belief in stereotypical media messages about women and/or sexual behaviors and attitudes [Ward, Merriwether, & Caruthers, 2006]. This is an area of research that should be explored in future media and gender studies with Black youth.

Racial Identity. One dimension of racial identity was associated with Black media images. Positive media images were negatively correlated with Private Regard. Initially, this finding appeared surprising; however in reality it is logical. Participants were asked to indicate how often they see images that reflect the selected messages on TV. Overall youth reported lower frequencies of viewing television images that projected positive messages. It is possible youth with higher Private Regard scores scrutinize media images and would be less inclined to ascribe positive messages to media images.

In contrast, youth who are high in Public Regard believe that the general public positively views Black people as a racial group. As such, they are less likely to identify the images of Black people in the public media as negative, even if they might be. In a sense, racial identity is like a pair of glasses that tends to highlight or play down some aspects in the media context. High Public Regard students report experiencing less racial discrimination and are less likely to see being Black as a central part of their identity [Arrington & Stevenson, 2006, 2007].

Body Image. Body image is very much influenced by socially accepted norms. Mainstream definitions of beauty rarely consider or include Black women [Patton, 2006]. However, because this study is about media images of Black people, we expected there would be a relationship between media images and body image, but when all four body image variables were entered into a correlation matrix with the media variables, none of the relationships were significant. This result could be an effect of cultural preference – viewing Black women who may share similar physical features to the youth or someone they know, and an acceptance of larger body types in the Black community. Alleyne and LaPoint's [2004] study suggests Black women and girls' tolerance for so-called large-size women may have evolved from West African standards of beauty [Alleyne & LaPoint, 2004]. Additional research with Black female youth about body ideals and body image within the Black community will help researchers to better understand how and whether Black media exposure relates to their body image ideals.

For the most part research interventions operate on the implicit assumption that being overweight is unfavorable. As such, these types of interventions are less likely to have an impact on health and lifestyle choice for Black girls who do not share this perspective. Further, Black media images that reinforce unhealthy eating and marketing strategies that use Black actors to advertise fast food and advertise poor food selections during peak viewing for Black audiences likely contribute to the eating habits of Black youth [Bertrand, 2002; Jacobs Henderson & Baldasty, 2003]. Research interventions for Black youth that are designed to encourage healthy lifestyle choices should consider the impact of Black media and how to influence behavior and attitude change with Black youth without totally negating cultural strengths and traditions.

Racial Socialization. It was expected that youth with higher R/E socialization scores would identify significantly more positive messages about Black people when watching TV; however, as demonstrated, this hypothesis was not supported. It may be that youth with higher R/E socialization scores are unlikely to identify positive messages about Black people when watching TV if in fact those positive images and messages are not prevalent on TV.

Despite the lack of significant findings for CARES variables, we believe the entire adolescent development process for Black youth is shaped by their R/E socialization experience, which in turn influences their perception of the world and their identity. Stevenson argues that racial identity is a mediating influence on identity development for Black adolescents, but that R/E experiences influence racial identity and that both are influences but do not mediate development in the same way [Stevenson, 2011]. While a significant relationship between N-BMMB scores and the CARES Stereotype and Racialism factors was not found, future research might consider increasing the sample size to re-examine these relationships[12].

Self-Esteem. The RSE measure was incorporated into this study because it is a commonly accepted instrument for assessing self-esteem. We hypothesized there would be a significant relationship between the youth with high self-esteem scores

---

[12] Though exploratory regression analyses were not reported, CARES factors were individually very close to being related but approaching significance ($p < 0.07$, 0.08, 0.13, etc.) with the BMMQ and SATAQ-3 factors in these models. This suggests that the results were affected by size of the sample.

and the BMMQ variables. However, like prior research, our study demonstrated that Black youth score high on this measure. Limiting the definition of global esteem to how one is perceived by others provides very little insight into the esteem of Black youth. The results of this study demonstrate that researchers who continue to investigate the esteem of Black youth using this methodology will continue to misinterpret the high self-esteem scores of Black adolescents and miss opportunities to develop intervention and/or treatment models that are inclusive of and appropriately address the developmental challenges of Black youth.

Theoretical Paradigms: Media Research and Black Adolescents
Cultivation Theory. Cultivation theory is understood to cultivate the dominant tendencies of a culture's beliefs, ideologies, and worldviews. Theoretically, the United States is governed by a singular set of beliefs and perspectives. Realistically, national ideologies of fair, just, and equitable treatment of all citizens do not fully translate into how institutions (industry) function and how people interact with one another. The media industry is an integral element of American society wherein racial, cultural, and gender biases persist in the media products produced. Television images of Black people are frequently controlled and/or created by non-Black entities that present stereotypical characterizations [Allen & Thornton, 1992].

In Stereotypes in the Media: So What? Gorham suggests racial stereotypes in the media are important contributors to racial myths, which are sustained via repeated exposure. As a result these myths inform how individuals process subsequent information about the group or individual being stereotyped [Gorham, 1999]. Our critique of cultivation theory is that it does not explicitly incorporate the perspective or intentions of the people responsible for creating the images. Instead, cultivation theory implies that television media is designed for entertainment. Thus researchers

approach the effects of media exposure as incidental to the utility of viewing TV and using other media for entertainment.

Ecological Media Research. In 2000, Berry wrote *Multicultural Media Portrayals and the Changing Demographic Landscape: The Psychosocial Impact of Television Representations on the Adolescent of Color*, which summarized media research with adolescents and critiqued common research platforms for the failure to consider how media influences work to manipulate adolescent development within the context of youth's familial and community environment(s) [Berry, 2000]. He suggested researchers take an 'ecological media research approach'. This approach uses mixed methods to study the cognitive and emotional effects of new media forms within a context of the culture of the youth, not apart from the important roots of the home and family [Berry, 2000]. Similar to PVEST, which allows for contextual analysis of behavior, this approach recognizes that the researcher must appreciate the intercultural variability found in minority groups so that the predictor variables and other parts of the design do not rely on preconceived and faulty views about youth of color [Berry, 2000]. From the authors' perspective, the five ecological media research questions Berry proposes for consideration when designing research models conflict with the implicit principles of cultivation theory.

Education Entertainment Theory (EET). We suggest researchers consider Education Entertainment Theory (EET) as a conceptual framework. EET[13] proposes that repeated exposure to a well-crafted media message affects attitude and behavioral change. Attitude and behavioral changes are elements of racial identity and racial socialization experience. Researchers who use EET intentionally create culturally driven media products, TV shows, radio shows, magazines,

[13] Theories mapping the underlying psychological processes and effects of entertainment-education programs are borrowed and adapted from traditional persuasion theories and models of health belief changes [Singhal & Rogers, 2002].

etc. that are designed to influence attitude and behavior. These mechanisms are mostly used for public health campaigns. Well-known campaigns against smoking, alcoholic use during pregnancy, and HIV/AIDS have proven successful at influencing behavior change and attitude [Singhal & Rogers, 2002]. Both an asset and weakness, EET is a conglomeration of marketing, psychological, and social theories, both qualitative and quantitative, that have proven effective particularly with repeated exposure [Slater & Rouner, 2002]. However, this paradigm has stimulated two major critiques of EET.

The first critique is that the combination of multiple disciplines makes it difficult for researchers to isolate, quantify, and capture the effects of projects that are designed using this theory. The second critique is aimed at the longitudinal design of EET studies, which typically rely on progressive increased exposure via message saturation through multiple media outlets. These studies occur over time, relying on repeated exposure to the media product(s) to initiate discourse and influence attitude and behavior among those who have been exposed to the campaigns [Brown, 2000; Slater & Rouner, 2002]. Opponents of EET argue that this design does not account for external factors that influence attitude and behavior change. They argue that significant or sustained attitude and behavior changes may not be the result of campaign exposure; historical moments in time, community level change, relationships, and developmental changes may be as influential as the media campaigns.

The authors acknowledge the shortcomings of EET, but reference the documented success of the EET campaigns mentioned above as evidence that sustained EET-driven initiatives have been proven to change behavior and influence attitudes. We believe the persistent portrayals of Black people as stereotypically negative are archetypologies in the media and that these typologies are an intentional extension of the historic and sociocultural role racism plays in American society, media images are designed to reinforce negative perceptions of Black people.

An EET theoretical framework would explicitly acknowledge the intent of the media producers. By doing so, researchers would have an opportunity to measure the effectiveness of the media for meeting the producer's goals through the development of an integrative research design. In turn, this would allow researchers to address Berry's five questions: (1) To what extent are the hate messages, images, and values available on the Internet having a negative effect on the youth of the racial and religious groups being targeted or identified, as well as on the cross-cultural attitudes and behaviors of the non-minority youth who must grow, develop, and function in an increasingly multicultural society? (2) What will be the educational, social, economic/career, and psychological/emotional impact on those youth who will have limited access to the new media; what of the lack of equity associated with the new technologies? (3) What are the historical, economic, political, and personal worldviews and belief systems that guide the decision-making processes inside the media industry that result in the lack of multicultural images and stories and continued stereotypes in the media? (4) Can schema theory help explain how youth of color and White Americans process, learn, and comprehend ethnic content? (5) What is the potential of multiethnic programs, games, and other new media to produce characters who will be able to enhance self-esteem, influence achievement motivation, reduce stereotypes, and function as positive cross-cultural role models for all adolescents [Berry, 2000]?

PVEST. These five questions can be addressed within the PVEST framework [Spencer, 2006]. For example, a researcher could use PVEST to frame question 2, defining and identifying the variables to be measured, determining which should be protective or risk factors or supports and challenges to select assessment strategies and measurements for a media research study with Black adolescents that provides answers to this inquiry. Berry's questions are inclusive of newer media technologies and can be applied to traditional mediums such as television, magazines, and radio. Essentially, combining the theoretical strengths of EET and PVEST to conduct ecological media research would provide us with clearer, more insightful answers about how exposure to negative media influences the identity processes of Black adolescents.

Implications for Future Research

This is an exploratory study. However, the results presented offer both a foundation and a pathway for conducting research with Black adolescents that incorporate Black media images and include R/E socialization and racial identity. Research with Black samples that focuses on media designed for Black audiences or incorporates context variables demonstrates a qualitative difference in outcomes when judged against comparative studies. Unfortunately, few studies with Black youth actually incorporate racial socialization into the design and analysis.

Age and gender were key indicators of whether youth identify negative stereotype messages and whether they endorse them. As noted earlier, body image and self-esteem studies rarely provide insight into the Black media images as influential on the body image and self-esteem of Black youth. This finding could be used to conduct pilot studies with Black youth about Black media images and body image to formulate a Black body image measure for incorporation into future studies.

The findings of this study also suggest endorsement of negative stereotype images on TV and to a lesser extent in magazines are impacted by the racial identity and racial socialization of Black adolescents. Our study like the few existing studies that include these two variables demonstrates that they are salient to the adolescent identity process of Black youth. Further, this study, unlike most media studies with adolescents focused exclusively on Black media images. Given the media preferences of Black youth to view shows with majority Black casts and the prevalence of Black media stereotypes, researchers should be sure to include Black media images in future studies. Although there were no significant relationships among the media variables and self esteem, there were significant relationships among the racial identity and media variables. Both racial identity and self-esteem are measures of self-concept; perhaps future media studies should examine how these variables relate to each other and determine if together they provide insight into how media influences the Black adolescent identity development process.

Acknowledgements

The empirical research presented in this chapter is taken from the dissertation study of the first author.

This research was supported in part by a grant from the Ruth Landes Memorial Research Fund, a program of The Reed Foundation.

References

Adams, V.N. (2009). *Black Media Messages Questionnaire (BMMQ)*. Psychological Questionnaire. Philadelphia: University of Pennsylvania.

Adams, V.N., & Stevenson, H.C. (2011). *Measuring Black media stereotypes.* Ithaca: Cornell University.

Allen, R.L., & Bielby, W.T. (1977). *Blacks' Attitudes and Behaviors Toward Television.* Paper presented at the Association for Education in Journalism, Madison.

Allen, R.L., & Bielby, W.T. (1979). Blacks' attitudes and behaviors toward television. *Communication Research, 6,* 437–462.

Allen, R.L., & Thornton, M.C. (1992). Social structural factors, black media and stereotypical self-characterization among African Americans. *National Journal of Sociology,* 41–75.

Alleyne, S.I., & LaPoint, V. (2004). Obesity among Black adolescent girls: Genetic, psychosocial, and cultural influences. *Journal of Black Psychology, 30,* 344–365.

Arnett, J.J. (1995). Adolescents' uses of media for self-socialization. *Journal of Youth & Adolescence, 24.*

Arnett, J.J., Larson, R., & Offer, D. (1995). Beyond effects: Adolescents as active media users. *Journal of Youth and Adolescence, 24,* 511–518.

Arrington, E.G., & Stevenson, H.C. (2006). Success of African American Students in Independent Schools: Final Report I. (G.S.o.E. Applied Psychology and Human Development, Trans.). Philadelphia: University of Pennsylvania.

Arrington, E.G., & Stevenson, H.C. (2007). Success of African American Students in Independent Schools: Final Report II. (G.S.o.E. Applied Psychology and Human Development, Trans.). Philadelphia: University of Pennsylvania.

Balaji, M. (2008). Vixen resistin': Redefining Black womanhood in hip-hop music videos. *Journal of Black Studies.* doi: 10.1177/0021934708325377.

Balaji, M. (2009). Why do good girls have to be bad?: The cultural industry's production of the other and the complexities of agency. *Popular Communication: The International Journal of Media and Culture, 7,* 225–236.

Bandura, A., Ross, D., & Ross, S.A. (1963). Imitation of film-mediated aggressive models. *Journal of Abnormal and Social Psychology, 66,* 3–11.

Barr, S.C., & Neville, H.A. (2008). Examination of the link between parental racial socialization messages and racial ideology among Black college students. *Journal of Black Psychology, 34,* 131–155. doi: 10.1177/0095798408314138.

Bentley, K.L., Adams, V.N., & Stevenson, H.C. (2009). Racial socialization: Roots, processes, and outcomes. In H. Neville, B. Tynes & S. Utsey (Eds.), *Handbook of African American Psychology* (pp. 258–267). Thousand Oaks: Sage Publications, Inc.

Bentley, K.L., & Stevenson, H.C. (2011). Beyond pride and mothers: Recasting racial/ethnic socialization measurement for multidimensional processes and informants.

Berry, G.L. (1998). Black family life on television and the socialization of the African American child: Images of marginality. *Journal of Comparative Family Studies, 29,* 233–242.

Berry, G.L. (2000). Multicultural media portrayals and the changing demographic landscape: The psychosocial impact of television representations on the adolescent of color. *Journal of Adolescent Health, 27S,* 57–60.

Bertrand, D. (2002). Black TV shows send unhealthy food messages. *Journal of National Medical Association, 94,* A9.

Bickham, D.S., Vandewater, E.A., Huston, A.C., Lee, J.H., Caplovitz, A.G., & Wright, J.C. (2003). Predictors of children's electronic media use: An examination of three ethnic groups. *Media Psychology, 5,* 107–137.

Biocca, F.A. (1988). Opposing conceptions of the audience: The active and passive hemispheres of mass communication theory. In J.A. Anderson (Ed.), *Communication Yearbook. Vol. 11* (pp. 51–80). Beverly Hills: Sage Publications, Inc.

Blosser, B.J. (1988). Ethnic differences in children's media use. *Journal of Broadcasting and Electronic Media, 32,* 453–470.

Bogle, D. (1973). Toms, Coons, Mulattoes, Mammies & Bucks: An interpretive history of Blacks in American films. New York: Bantam Books.

Bogle, D. (1980). Brown sugar: Eighty years of American Black female superstars. New York: Da Capo Press.

Bogle, D. (2001a). Primetime blues: African Americans on network television. New York: Fararr, Straus & Giroux.

Bogle, D. (2001b). Toms, Coons, Mulattoes, Mammies & Bucks: An interpretive history of Blacks in American films (4th ed.). New York: Continuum International Publishing Group.

Brown, B., & Marin, P. (2009). Adolescents and electronic media: Growing up plugged in. *Trends Child Research Brief* (pp. 1–11). Washington, DC: Child Trends and the National Adolescent Health Information Center.

Brown, J.D. (2000). Adolescents' sexual media diets. *Journal of Adolescent Health, 27*(2, Supplement 1), 35–40.

Browne Graves, S. (1982). The impact of television on the cognitive and affective development of minority children. In G.L. Berry & C. Mitchell-Kernan (Eds.), *Television and the socialization of the minority child* (pp. 42–67). New York: Academic Press.

Bush, A.J., Smith, R., & Martin, C. (1999). The influence of consumer socialization variables on attitude toward advertising: A comparison of African-Americans and Caucasians. *Journal of Advertising, 28,* 13–24.

Calvert, S.l. (2008). Children as consumers: Advertising and marketing. *The Future of Children, 18,* 205–234.

Coltrane, S., & Messineo, M. (2000). The perpetuation of subtle prejudice: Race and gender imagery in 1990s television advertising. *Sex Roles, 42,* 363–389.

Davis, J.L., & Gandy, O.H. (1999). Racial identity and media orientation: Exploring the nature of constraint. *Journal of Black Studies, 29,* 367–397.

Escobar-Chaves, S.L., & Anderson, C.A. (2008). Media and risky behaviors. *The Future of Children, 18,* 147–180.

Evans, W.D. (2008). Social marketing and children's media use. *The Future of Children, 18, 181–204.*

Fujioka, Y. (2005). Black media images as a perceived threat to African American ethnic identity: Coping responses, perceived public perception, and attitudes towards affirmative action. *Journal of Broadcasting & Electronic Media, 49,* 450–467.

Gerbner, G. (1998). Cultivation analysis: An overview. *Mass Communication and Society, 1,* 175–194.

Gerbner, G., & Gross, L. (1976). Living with television: The violence profile. *Journal of Communication, 26,* 172–194.

Gordon, M.K. (2008). Media contributions to African American girls' focus on beauty and appearance: Exploring the consequences of sexual objectification. *Psychology of Women Quarterly, 32,* 245–256.

Gorham, B.W. (1999). Stereotypes in the media: So what? *The Harvard Journal of Communications, 10,* 229–247.

Grier, S., & Bryant, C.A. (2005). Social marketing in public health. *Annual Review of Public Health, 26,* 319–339.

Heide, M.J. (1995). Television culture and women's lives: Thirty something and the contradictions of gender. Philadelphia: University of Pennsylvania Press.

Hughes, D., Rodriguez, J., Smith, E.P., Johnson, D.J., Stevenson, H.C., & Spicer, P. (2006). Parents' ethnic-racial socialization practices: A review of research and directions for future study. *Developmental Psychology, 42,* 747–770.

Jackson, R.L. (2006). Scripting the Black masculine body identity, discourse, and racial politics in popular media. Albany: State University of New York Press.

Jacobs Henderson, J., & Baldasty, G.J. (2003). Race, advertising, and prime-time television. *The Harvard Journal of Communications, 14,* 97.

Jefferson, R.S. (1970). A critique of syndicated television and its effect on black people. *Journal of the National Medical Association, 62,* 122–128.

Lee, E.B., & Browne, L.A. (1981). Television uses and gratifications among Black children, teenagers, and adults. *Journal of Broadcasting, 25,* 203–208.

McQuail, D. (2005). *McQuail's mass communication theory* (5th ed.). London: Sage Publications, Inc.

Nama, A. (2003). More symbol than substance: African American representation in network television dramas. *Race and Society, 6,* 21–38.

O'Connor, L.A., Brooks-Gunn, J., & Graber, J. (2000). Black and White Girls' racial preferences in media and peer choices and the role of socialization for Black girls. *Journal of Family Psychology, 14,* 510–521.

Parker, D. (1999). *Thinking critically about the messages of the media: Female images and roles.* Doctoral Dissertation, University of Illinois at Urbana-Champaign, Urbana-Champaign.

Patton, T.O. (2006). Hey Girl, Am I More than My Hair?: African American women and their struggles with beauty, body image, and hair. *NWSA (National Women's Studies Association) Journal, 18,* 24–51.

Plomin, R., Foch, T.T., & Rowe, D.C. (1981). Bobo clown aggression in childhood: Environment, not genes. *Journal of Research in Personality, 15,* 331–342.

Ramasubramanian, S. (2007). Media-based strategies to reduce racial stereotypes activated by news stories. *Journalism and Mass Communication Quarterly, 84,* 249–264.

Roberts, D.F., & Foehr, U.G. (2008). Trends in media use. *The Future of Children, 18,* 11–38.

Rosenberg, M. (1989). *Society and the adolescent self-image (Rev.ed.).* Middletown: Wesleyan University Press.

Scottham, K.M., Sellers, R.M., & Nguyên, H.X. (2008). A measure of racial identity in African American adolescents: The development of the Multidimensional Inventory of Black Identity–Teen. *Cultural Diversity and Ethnic Minority Psychology, 14,* 297–306.

Singhal, A., & Rogers, E.M. (2002). A theoretical agenda for Entertainment-Education. *Communication Theory, 12,* 117–135.

Slater, M.S., & Rouner, D. (2002). Entertainment-Education and elaboration likelyhood: Understanding the processing of narrative persuasion. *Communication Theory, 12,* 173–191.

Spencer, M.B. (1995). Old issues and new theorizing about African-American youth: A phenomenological variant of ecological systems theory. In R.L. Taylor (Ed.), *African American youth: Their social and economic status in the United States* (pp. 37–69). Westport: Praeger.

Spencer, M.B. (2006). Phenomenology and ecological systems theory: Development of diverse groups. In W. Damon & R. Lerner (Eds.), *Handbook of child psychology theoretical models of human development. Vol. 1* (6th ed., pp. 829–893). New York: Wiley.

Spencer, M.B., Dupree, D., Swanson, D.P., & Cunningham, M. (1996). Parental monitoring and adolescents' sense of responsibility for their own learning: An examination of sex differences. *Journal of Negro Education, 65,* 30–43.

Stevenson, H.C. (2011). Recasting racially anxious encounters theorizing racial/ethnic coping and agency socialization. Philadelphia: University of Pennsylvania.

Stevenson, H.C., & Arrington, E.G. (2009). Racial/ethnic socialization mediates perceived racism and the racial identity of African American adolescents. *Cultural Diversity and Ethnic Minority Psychology, 15,* 125–136.

Strasburger, V.C., Wilson, B.J., & Jordan, A.B. (2009). Children and adolescents: Unique audiences. In C. Dellelo & E. Evans (Eds.), *Children, adolescents, and the media* (2nd ed., pp. 1–35). Thousand Oaks: Sage Publications, Inc.

Stroman, C.A. (1991). Television's role in the socialization of African American children and adolescents. *Journal of Negro Education, 60,* 314–327.

Thompson, J.K., Patricia, V.D.B., Roehrig, M., Guarda, A.S., & Heinberg, L.J. (2004). The Sociocultural Attitudes Towards Appearance Scale-3 (SATAQ-3): Development and validation. *International Journal of Eating Disorders, 35,* 293–304.

Tynes, B.M., & Ward, L.M. (2009). The role of media use and portrayals in African Americans' psychosocial development. In H.A. Neville, B.M. Tynes & S.O. Utsey (Eds.), *Handbook of African American Psychology* (pp. 143–158). Thousand Oaks: Sage Publications, Inc.

Vercellotti, T., & Brewer, P.R. (2006). 'To Plead Our Own Cause': Public opinion toward Black and mainstream news media among African Americans. *Journal of Black Studies, 37,* 231–250.

Walsh, D.C., Rudd, R.E., Moeykens, B.A., & Moloney, T.W. (1993). Social marketing for public health. *Health Affairs, 12,* 104–119.

Ward, L.M. (2004). Wading through the stereotypes: Positive and negative associations between media use and Black adolescents' conceptions of self. *Developmental Psychology, 40,* 284–294.

Ward, L.M., Day, K.M., & Epstein, M. (2006). Uncommonly good: Exploring how mass media may be a positive influence on young women's sexual health and development. *New Directions for Child and Adolescent Development, 112,* 57–70.

Ward, L.M., Hansbrough, E., & Walker, E. (2005). Contributions of music video exposure to Black adolescents' gender and sexual schemas. *Journal of Adolescent Research, 20,* 143–166.

Ward, L.M., Merriwether, A., & Caruthers, A. (2006). Breasts are for men: Media, masculinity ideologies, and men's beliefs about women's bodies. *Sex Roles, 55,* 703–714.

Wartella, E., O'Keefe, B., & Scantlin, R. (2000). Children and interactive media: A compendium of current research and directions for the future (p. 195). New York, NY: The Markle Foundation.

Watkins, S.C. (2000). Black youth and mass media: Current research and emerging questions. *African American Research Perspectives*, 6. Retrieved April 22, 2005 from http://rcgd.isr.umich.edu/prba/perspectives/winter2000/cwatkins.pdf.

Woodard, J.B., & Mastin, T. (2005). Black womanhood: Essence and its treatment of stereotypical images of Black women. *Journal of Black Studies, 36*, 264–281.

Dr. Valerie N. Adams (PhD 2011, Applied Psychology and Human Development, University of Pennsylvania) is the New York State 4-H Program Leader at the Bronfenbrenner Center for Translational Research and Assistant Director of Cooperative Extension at Cornell University. Her research interests are how racial socialization and racial identity influence the identity development process of African American adolescents. Her research also investigates how racial socialization and racial identity relate to the interpretation of stereotyped Black media images and what relationships exists between exposure to these images and the body image and self esteem of Black youth.

Dr. Howard C. Stevenson (PhD, Fuller Graduate School of Psychology) is Associate Professor of Education and a member of the Applied Psychology and Human Development Division in the Graduate School of Education at the University of Pennsylvania. His research interests include the development of theory, measurement, and interventions on racial/ethnic socialization as a mediator of racial stress for youth and families. He is a co-editor with Diana Slaughter-Defoe of *Black Educational Choice: Assessing the Private and Public Alternatives to K-12 Public Schools* [Praeger, 2011], editor of *Playing with anger: Teaching coping skills to African American boys through athletics and culture* [Praeger, 2003], and co-author with Gwendolyn Davis and Saburah Abdul-Kabir of *Stickin' to, watchin' over, and getting' with: An African American parent's guide to discipline* [Jossey-Bass, 2001].

Valerie N. Adams
Bronfenbrenner Center for Translational Research, Cornell University
125 Plantations Road
Ithaca, NY 14850 (USA)
Tel. +1 607 255 7958
E-Mail vnadams1@gmail.com

Commentary

Slaughter-Defoe DT (ed): Racial Stereotyping and Child Development.
Contrib Hum Dev. Basel, Karger, 2012, vol 25, pp 47–51

Adolescents, Race, and Media

Commentary on Adams and Stevenson

Jessica Taylor Piotrowski

Center for Research on Children, Adolescents, and the Media (CCAM), Amsterdam School of Communication Research (ASCoR), University of Amsterdam, Amsterdam, The Netherlands

Adams and Stevenson investigate how the stereotypical portrayals of Blacks in the media are associated with Black adolescents' endorsements of these images. They find that the endorsements of negative stereotypes are not universal, but rather are dependent upon individual characteristics of the adolescent. From a communication paradigm, there are several strengths to their research. First, their work recognizes the powerful role that media play in adolescents' lives. Second, rather than focus solely on quantity, the researchers acknowledge that media quality is critical to evaluating media effects. And lastly, by recognizing the role of the media consumer, they recognize the cyclical process of media effects. Their research highlights two key questions that researchers should ask when studying how media affect adolescents: (1) What do media bring to adolescents? and (2) What do adolescents bring to media?

What Do Media Bring to Adolescents?

Adolescents spend nearly 8 hours per day engaging with media [Rideout, Foehr & Roberts, 2010], making it a powerful force in their lives. The messages they consume from media affect them in diverse ways. Exposure to violent media content has been linked to subsequent aggressive behavior [Huesmann, Moise-Titus, Podolski & Eron, 2003] while exposure to sexualized media content has been linked with sexual behavior [Bleakley, Hennessy, Fishbein & Jordan, 2008]. Media can also support adolescents' healthy development. Depicting consequences of unprotected sex encourages adolescents to speak with their parents about condom use [Collins, Elliott, Berry, Kanouse & Hunter, 2003], anti-tobacco messages decrease smoking initiation among adolescents [Siegel & Biener, 2002], and realistic depictions of women can counter body dissatisfaction among adolescent females [Halliwell, Easun & Harcourt, 2011]. Adolescents do learn from media and the content of the media matters.

Although the societal concern about media effects typically focuses upon behavior [Ward, 2005], Adams & Stevenson's research reminds us that media also contribute to beliefs about ourselves and others – including racial beliefs. In our highly segregated society, the opportunity to interact with people of another racial group remains limited – particularly for White youth [Frey & Myers, 2002; Ward, 2005]. Media, thought to be our most common and constant learning environment [Morgan, 2007], often provide the most regular 'contact' with individuals from other racial groups [Ward, 2005]. Repeated contact with the media, according to cultivation theorists, will eventually shape people's beliefs and assumptions of the real world so that their beliefs mirror the media's depictions [Gerbner, Gross, Morgan, Signorielli & Shanahan, 2002]. Adolescents' susceptibility to external influences combined with their limited real-world experiences make them highly susceptible to cultivation effects [Morgan, 2007].

Media provide information about racial groups in one of two ways: by inclusion and by exclusion [Graves, 1999]. Content analyses indicate that non-Whites are underrepresented in the media, and are more likely to be cast in minor roles [Children Now, 2004; Gilmore & Jordan, in press]. While inroads have been made in children's programs [Bramlett-Solomon & Roeder, 2008; Calvert, Stolkin & Lee, 1997] and in prime-time media for Black characters [Mastro, 2009], underrepresentation remains. This exclusion teaches adolescents that non-Whites are unimportant and inconsequential [Graves, 1999; Van Evra, 2004; Vittrup & Holden, 2010]. Equally concerning, when included in the media, non-Whites are often presented in negative or stereotypical ways sending the message that non-Whites are criminals, lazy, aggressive, and financially insecure [Berry, 2007; Dixon & Linz, 2002; Ward, 2005] as well as promoting the view that they lack power and status [Vittrup & Holden, 2010]. For White adolescents, these inaccurate and negative portrayals can cultivate in-group favoritism at the expense of out-group tolerance [Vittrup & Holden, 2010] making adolescents more likely to become prejudiced adults. Research has in fact shown that frequent exposure to stereotypical portrayals of Blacks leads to a greater endorsement of these stereotypes and more negative attitudes towards Blacks in general [Lee, Bichard, Irey, Walt & Carlson, 2009; Ramasubramanian, 2010].

The effect of such inaccurate portrayals is clearly of concern for White adolescents, but how might these portrayals affect non-White adolescents? This question is especially important given that Black and Latino youths consume significantly more media than their White counterparts [Rideout, Lauricella & Wartella, 2011] and thus are more vulnerable to its portrayals of race [Ward, 2005]. By virtue of underrepresentation and misrepresentation, non-White adolescents will likely feel unimportant, inconsequential, and powerless [Stroman, 1991] which can lead to poorer self-esteem. Research with Black adolescents supports this contention with higher rates of media exposure associated with lower self-esteem [Ward, 2004]. This association is tempered by a host of factors. For example, although the omnibus findings demonstrate a negative association, stronger identification with popular Black characters is associated with higher self-esteem for Black adolescents while stronger identification with White characters is associated with lower self-esteem [Ward, 2004]. This suggests that there may be protective factors that non-White adolescents can employ when using media, and underscores the importance of understanding what adolescents bring to media.

What Do Adolescents Bring to Media?

Although the general public seems to accept that media have powerful, direct effects on individuals, most media effects scholars disagree [Oliver & Krakowiak, 2009]. Adolescents do not approach media as blank slates, rather they bring with them experiences which shape how they use media and how media affects them. Ecological theory [Bronfenbrenner & Morris, 1998] posits that adolescents develop within a series of nested environments ranging from their daily experiences (microsystem; e.g. home or school life), to interactions across these daily experiences (mesosystem), to the institutions that indirectly impact them (exosystem; e.g. parental employment) to the larger cultural context in which they are developing (macrosystem; e.g. race). These systems influence how adolescents approach and use media [Jordan, 2004, 2005]. For example, compared to White adolescents, Black and Hispanic youth are more likely to have a television in their bedroom, to eat more meals with the television on, and to live in homes where the television is always on [Rideout et al., 2011]. Growing up in such distinct microsystems where television has different structural and relational uses [Lull, 1980], it is fair to expect that Black and Hispanic youth will approach television differently than White youth. And in fact, extant research [see Ward, 2004] does suggest that Black youth approach television differently by holding more favorable attitudes towards television, reporting higher levels of satisfaction with television, and more frequently using television for information and guidance.

By evaluating Black adolescents' interpretation of media images of Black people in the context of individual differences, Adams and Stevenson are acknowledging that the effects of media are not monolithic. Moreover, their decision to develop a tailored assessment tool for work with Black adolescents reflects an effort to better understand how the macrosystem of race impacts adolescents' experiences with media. They find that youth who have a higher private regard – a dimension of racial identity reflecting a confidence in one's race – were more likely to assert that positive messages associated with Black images were accurate, and were less likely to agree with negative statements associated with Black images. They also found that youth who have a deeper racial socialization (the ability to guard against racially stressful encounters as well as an ability

to uphold and support the experiences of Black people) are more likely to believe positive media messages about Black people. While experimental research is needed to confirm causal order as well as replications with other non-White populations, these findings suggest that efforts to enhance the racial identity of non-White youth may be worthwhile as they seem to offer some protection from negative presentations in the media. The work also suggests that supporting the development of adolescents' racial identity and racial socialization may provide them with tools to capitalize on the less frequent, but available, positive media portrayals.

Concluding Thoughts

Greater, more diverse portrayals of non-Whites are critical for the healthy development of adolescents. Media have the ability to be an excellent tool for teaching and learning in a growing multicultural landscape such as the United States [Berry, 2007]. To that end, media developers must make efforts to ensure that they are providing culturally balanced images. These media images should be crafted from an 'emic perspective that looks at groups from within their own cultural framework as opposed to the etic perspective that views people through the comparative lens outside of their culture' [Berry, 2007, p. 104]. In doing so, we can harness the cultivation power of the media to help adolescents understand and value themselves and others.

Researchers must also recognize that interpretation of media content is dependent on individual differences. Adams and Stevenson, for example, show how select individual differences can serve as protective factors for Black adolescents against the negative stereotypes present within the media. More broadly, their work evidences the importance of contributing within-group analyses to the scholarly conversation on adolescents, race, and media. Adolescents bring with them a host of experiences which shape how they use media and how it affects them – with race being a global macrostructure that informs this socialization. If our aim is to support the development of culturally aware adolescents, our research designs and methods must reflect this aim.

References

Berry, G.L. (2007). Television, social roles, and marginality: Portrayals of the past and images for the future. In N. Pecora, J.P. Murray & E. Wartella (Eds.), *Children and television: Fifty years of research* (pp. 85–107). Mahwah: Lawrence Erlbaum.

Bleakley, A., Hennessy, M., Fishbein, M., & Jordan, A. (2008). It works both ways: The relationship between exposure to sexual content in the media and adolescent sexual behavior. *Media Psychology, 11*, 443–461.

Bramlett-Solomon, S., & Roeder, Y. (2008). Looking at race in children's television. *Journal of Children and Media, 2,* 56–66. doi: 10.1080/17482790701 733187.

Bronfenbrenner, U., & Morris, P. (1998). The ecology of developmental processes. In W. Damon & N. Eisenberg (Eds.), *Handbook of child psychology. Vol. 1: Ch. 17* (5th ed., pp. 993–1028). New York: Wiley.

Calvert, S.L., Stolkin, A., & Lee, J. (1997). Gender and ethnic portrayals in Saturday morning television programs. Poster presented at the biennial meeting of the *Society for Research in Child Development*. Washington, DC. (ERIC Document Reproduction Service No. ED407119).

Children Now. (2004). *Fall colors: Prime time diversity report 2003–04.* Oakland: Children Now.

Collins, R.L., Elliott, M.N., Berry, S.H., Kanouse, D.E., & Hunter, S.B. (2003). Entertainment television as a healthy sex educator: The impact of condom-efficacy information in an episode of Friends. *Pediatrics, 112,* 1115–1121.

Dixon, T.L., & Linz, D. (2002). Race and the misrepresentation of victimization on local television news. *Communication Research, 27,* 547–573.

Frey, W., & Myers, D. (2002). Neighborhood segregation in single-race and multi-race America: A census 2000 study of cities and metropolitan areas. Washington: Fannie Mae Foundation.

Gerbner, G., Gross, L., Morgan, M., Signorielli, N., & Shanahan, J. (2002). Growing up with television: Cultivation processes. In J. Bryant & D. Zillman (Eds.), *Media effects: Advances in theory and research* (pp. 43–67). Mahwah: Lawrence Erlbaum.

Gilmore, J.S., & Jordan, A. (in press). Burgers and basketball: Race and stereotypes in food/beverage advertising aimed at children in the U.S. *Journal of Children and Media.*

Graves, S.B. (1999). Television and prejudice reduction: When does television as a vicarious experience make a difference? *Journal of Social Issues, 55,* 707–725.

Halliwell, E., Easun, A., & Harcourt, D. (2011). Body dissatisfaction: Can a short media literacy message reduce negative media exposure effects amongst adolescent girls? *British Journal of Health Psychology, 16,* 396–403.

Huesmann, L.R., Moise-Titus, J., Podolski, C.L., & Eron, L.D. (2003). Longitudinal relations between children's exposure to TV violence and their aggressive and violent behavior in young adulthood. *Developmental Psychology, 39,* 201–221.

Jordan, A.B. (2004). The role of media in children's development: An ecological perspective. *Developmental and Behavioral Pediatrics, 25,* 196–206.

Jordan, A.B. (2005). Learning to use books and television. *American Behavioral Scientist, 48,* 525–538.

Lee, M.J., Bichard, S.L., Irey, M.S., Walt, H.M., & Carlson, A.J. (2009). Television viewing and ethnic stereotypes: Do college students form stereotypical perceptions of ethnic groups as a result of heavy television consumption? *The Howard Journal of Communications, 20,* 95–110.

Lull, J. (1980). The social uses of television. *Human Communication Research, 6,* 197–209.

Mastro, D. (2009). Effects of racial sterotyping and ethnic stereotyping. In J. Bryant & M.B. Oliver (Eds.), *Media effects: Advances in theory and research* (3rd ed.). New York: Lawrence Erlbaum.

Morgan, M. (2007). What do young people learn about the world from watching television? In S.R. Mazzarella (Ed.), *20 Questions about Youth and the Media* (pp. 153–166). New York: Peter Lang.

Oliver, M.B., & Krakowiak, K.M. (2009). Individual differences in media effects. In J. Bryant & M.B. Oliver (Eds.), *Media effects: Advances in theory and research* (3rd ed.). New York: Lawrence Erlbaum.

Ramasubramanian, S. (2010). Television viewing, racial attitudes, and policy preferences: Exploring the role of social identity and intergroup emotions in influencing support for affirmative action. *Communication Monographs, 77,* 102–120.

Rideout, V., Foehr, U.G., & Roberts, D.F. (2010). *Generation M2: Media in the lives of 8- to 18-year olds.* Menlo Park: Henry J. Kaiser Family Foundation.

Rideout, V., Lauricella, A.R., & Wartella, E. (2011). *Children, media, and race: Media use among White, Black, Hispanic, and Asian American children.* Evanston: Center on Media and Human Development, School of Communication, Northwestern University.

Siegel, M., & Biener, L. (2002). The impact of antismoking media campaigns on progression to established smoking: Results of a longitudinal youth study in Massachusetts. In R.C. Hornik (Ed.), *Public health communication: Evidence for behavior change* (pp. 115–130). Mahwah: Lawrence Erlbaum Associates.

Stroman, C.A. (1991). Television's role in the socialization of African American children and adolescents. *Journal of Negro Education, 60,* 314–327.

Van Evra, J. (2004). *Television and child development* (3rd ed.). Hillsdale: Lawrence Erlbaum Associates.

Vittrup, B., & Holden, G.W. (2010). Exploring the impact of educational television and parent-child discussions on children's racial attitudes. *Analyses of Social Issues and Public Policy, 10,* 192–214.

Ward, L.M. (2004). Wading through the stereotypes: Positive and negative associations between media use and black adolescents' conceptions of self. *Developmental Psychology, 40,* 284–294.

Ward, L.M. (2005). Children, adolescents, and the media: The molding of minds, bodies, and deeds. *New Directions for Child and Adolescent Development, 109,* 63–71.

Jessica Taylor Piotrowski, PhD
Center for Research on Children
Adolescents, and the Media (CCAM)
Amsterdam School of Communication
Research (ASCoR), University of Amsterdam
Kloveniersburgwal 48
NL–1012 CX Amsterdam (The Netherlands)
Tel. +31 (0) 20 525 3505
E-Mail j.piotrowski@uva.nl

Dr. Jessica Taylor Piotrowski (PhD 2010, Annenberg School for Communication, University of Pennsylvania) is an Assistant Professor in the Youth & Media Entertainment group in the Department of Communication Science at the University of Amsterdam. Her research focuses on understanding the role that media plays in the lives of young children. She views the individual differences of the viewer, the context of the media use, and the media content itself as equal contributors when evaluating media effects. Her research has been presented at numerous conferences and published in communication, psychology, and education journals.

Commentary

Slaughter-Defoe DT (ed): Racial Stereotyping and Child Development.
Contrib Hum Dev. Basel, Karger, 2012, vol 25, pp 52–54

Damned if You Do and Damned If You Don't! What are the Correct Media Images for Black People in the Media and How Can We Know?

Commentary on Adams and Stevenson

James M. Jones

Department of Psychology, University of Delaware, Newark, Del., USA

'The power of the media. . . is that it both reflects and creates images of [blacks] that lead to stereotypical perceptions and biasing expectation and behaviors. . .do [these stereotypical images] follow from the way society views blacks, or do they dictate how society will view blacks?' [Jones, 1997, p. 457].

Toms, Coons, mammies, Bucks, stepin fetchit, jezebels, sapphires, minstrels, Aunt Jemima are all images or characters in the portrayals of Black people in the media, mostly TV and movies. In the 1930s, the five most prevalent stereotypes of Black people, at least among Princeton men, were, in order; superstitious, lazy, happy-go-lucky, ignorant, musical [Katz & Braly, 1933, 1935]. However, Bayton et al. [1956] showed that these stereotypes were specific to lower class Blacks. Among Whites, upper class Blacks were stereotyped in order; intelligent, ambitious, ostentatious, industrious and courteous. It is not surprising that race and class may be confounded when we talk about stereotyping in the media. Further, it is likely that these effects are similarly variable as a function of the social class of the respondent.

Eugene Robinson [2010] argues that Black Americans have been splintered into four groups: (a) mainstream – comprised of the middle-class majority with a full ownership stake in American society; (b) emergent – comprised of individuals of mixed-race heritage and communities of recent Black immigrants; (c) transcendent – a small elite group with massive wealth, power and influence; and (d) abandoned – a minority with defeatist dreams and pessimistic hope. In the words of Robinson, '. . .these four black Americas are increasingly distinct, separated by demography, geography and psychology . . . leading separate lives' [Robinson, 2010, Chapter 1].

Media portrayals matter to be sure but how? Do viewers mistake fiction for reality? Or is the symbolism of semi-real portrayals so powerful that young Black children and adolescents adopt them as 'role models' to emulate? When Diahann Carrol played *Julia* in the 1960s, she was a nurse, a single parent and lived a middle class and racially integrated life. Her son, Cory, was 'informed' by his White playmate that he was colored. To which Cory replied, 'I am?' Julia was thought by many Blacks to be an 'inauthentic' portrayal of Black people [see Kleinman & Riggs, 1991; *Color adjustment* video]. Cosby came on the scene in the 1980s and portrayed a very middle class family that was undeniably Black. Yet they were criticized for being affluent. JJ was a minstrel in *Good Times*; President Obama is not 'black enough'.

What is the correct image to portray Black people? And which Black people are being portrayed and what do different strata of Black people want to see? What is positive to some is not to others and vice versa. Do they attach cultural meaning to the symbols, discern the hidden messages, and then accept or reject them depending on their level of racial socialization and racial identity? These are tough questions that, while they matter tremendously, are not at all easy to sort out.

For example, in the classic doll studies of Kenneth and Mamie Clark [1947], the children correctly identified the race of the dolls, but ascribed more positive qualities to the White dolls than the darker skinned dolls. Did they hate being Black, or did they understand the cultural meanings of Black and White and reflect that back to the examiners? It is not simple to go from an image to an identity, a portrayal to a principle.

Adams and Stevenson have made a valiant effort to address this thorny problem by bringing to bear conceptual tools and empirical procedures to its analysis. For this they must be applauded. Granting that it is difficult to know what causes what in this sort of analysis, and by and large, the data are self-report which makes it difficult to know what is really affecting what and what ideas get connected in a child's or adolescent's head, there are some important questions we need to ask.

First, study participants were not specified with regard to socioeconomic class. As we have seen that clearly makes a difference. They had participants evaluate 20 images on each of several different critical dependent measures but do not describe or depict the images. It would be really useful to know what images they used. How were they selected, and were they representative, and if so, of what? What stereotypes did they portray, and how subtle were they? A table of the correlations among the main variables would have helped

us follow the many pathways among the variables. Moreover, correlations tell us what is associated with what but does not allow us to weigh the relative strength of these associations of media understanding and perceptions on self-esteem, racial identity, socialization and so forth. A regression or structural equation analysis would be more informative of what is truly going on.

The authors make an important point about TV watching, so I wonder why they didn't focus on TV, or divide their sample into heavy and light TV viewing for the purposes of their analyses? They also mention other social media but did not assess that. They mentioned that interpretation and endorsement of Black media images would be mediated by racial socialization, Black history knowledge and self-esteem, but no mediational analyses were conducted. There are potentially 6 different mediational analyses implied by this statement.

Mediation tells us which mechanisms are mostly responsible for the associations among critical variables in a conceptual model. Moderation tells us whether the relationships we find are the same for different groups (say, different SES levels among Blacks; or age cohorts, etc.). And a mediated moderation analysis tells us that the mechanisms may work differently for different groups. As I have suggested, media images are complex in the Black community. Such analyses will be needed to tease apart the multiple impacts of sensitivity to, interpretation and influences of media images and messages on Black youth. Adams and Stevenson take an important step in that direction by conceptualizing some critical variables that must be better understood. Now future researchers need to provide a more comprehensive and complex analysis of these important variables.

Looking ahead, clearly we have not entered a post-racial America; rather the nature of racism is increasingly subtle, implicit, aversive, and postmodern. Thus media effects will be less transparent than they have been in the past. But they will still deliver messages that reinforce a racialized hierarchy of social values, self-worth, and power dynamics. Research will have to be more clever and more analytically complex to capture this growing subtlety and the multiple effects it can have on a range of Black youth.

It is also important to track media effects in longitudinal research designs. We know that context matters and socioeconomic status is a huge context for Black youth. Black youth in racially integrated suburban communities may be *more* prone to some subversive images, and *less* prone to others. The same could be said of middle and upper class Black youth compared to urban and rural poor Black youth. Not only is their socioeconomic status an important context, but very likely the socialization messages they receive from parents and peers, as well as their choice of media exposure may vary along these dimensions.

Finally, we need to ask how media images contribute to making the meaning Black youth find in their lives. It is likely that the images that prove the most impactful are those that share meanings that provide coherence and coping capacity. So the variables of racial identity [and perhaps we should add street-identity, after Payne, 2011], self-esteem, and probably more importantly life satisfaction and the meaning of life [see Ryff, 1989, for a good measure of life satisfaction] are certainly important to unraveling the impact of media messages and exposure on Black youth.

Adams and Stevenson have provided a good beginning. The years ahead are critical for advancing this work conceptually, methodologically and analytically.

References

Bayton, J.A., McAlister, L.B., & Hamer, J. (1956). Race-class stereotypes. *Journal of Negro Education, 41,* 75–78.

Clark, K.B., & Clark, M.P. (1947). Racial identification and preference in Negro children. In T.M. Newcomb & E.L. Hartley (Eds.), *Readings in social psychology* (1st ed.). New York: Holt.

Jones, J.M. (1997). *Prejudice and racism* (2nd ed.). New York: McGraw-Hill.

Katz, D., & Braly, K. (1933). Racial stereotypes of one hundred college students. *Journal of Abnormal and Social Psychology, 28,* 280–290.

Kleinman, V., & Riggs, M.T. (1991). *Color Adjustment (video).* San Francisco: California Newsreel.

Payne, Y.A. (2011). Site of resilience: A reconceptualization of resilience and resiliency in street life-oriented black men. *Journal of Black* Psychology, *37,* 426–451.

Robinson, E. (2010). Disintegration: The splintering of Black America. New York: Doubleday.

Ryff, C.D. (1989). Happiness is everything, or is it? Explorations on the meaning of psychological well-being. *Journal of Personality and Social Psychology, 57,* 1069–1081.

James M. Jones
Department of Psychology
University of Delaware
Newark, DE 19716 (USA)
Tel. +1 302 831 2489
E-Mail jmjones@psych.udel.edu

Dr. James M. Jones (PhD 1970, Yale University) is professor of psychology and Director of the Center for the Study of Diversity at the University of Delaware. His book, *Prejudice and racism,* was published initially in 1972 with a second edition in 1997. In addition to his writing on racism, he has written on the cultural psychology of blacks based on his TRIOS model and his concept of the Universal Context of Racism (UCR). TRIOSic people, as measured by his TRIOS scale, show resilience, a capacity to maintain positive psychological well-being and adaptive coping with racism. People high in the salience of racism as measured by his UCR construct, are vigilant about racism but if they do not have the TRIOS characteristics, they often suffer decreased psychological well-being.

Commentary

Slaughter-Defoe DT (ed): Racial Stereotyping and Child Development.
Contrib Hum Dev. Basel, Karger, 2012, vol 25, pp 55–56

Social Media, Privacy and Identity

Commentary on Adams and Stevenson

Andrea M. Matwyshyn

University of Pennsylvania, Philadelphia, Pa., USA

In Media Socialization, Black Media Images and Black Adolescent Identity, Valerie Adams and Howard Stephenson undertake an empirical examination of the relationships among exposure to negative stereotype Black media images, racial identity, racial socialization, body image and self-esteem for 14- to 21-year-old Black youth. Although the focus of their measures is on traditional media, they raise important questions regarding the impact of new media on Black adolescent identity.

In particular, the role of social media on adolescent identity warrants consideration. Adolescents are using social networks in record numbers: according to a recent Pew study, almost three quarters of online adolescents use social networks[1]. As such, social media are playing an increased role in the construction of identity for adolescents – both in terms of the content that adolescents post and in terms of the derivative information created by social networks about the adolescents.

Three important shifts away from traditional media paradigms are reflected in the dynamics of adolescents' use of social media. First, social networks progressively shift the information flows from visible intermediation to invisible intermediation. They change traditional media's uni-directional input to a bi-directional one: social media has shifted the 'push' dynamic of traditional media – a television show presenting certain types of images to the adolescent – to a 'push-pull' dynamic, where content evolves in a personalized manner. Adolescents now interact with companies and each other in real time and obtain instant feedback on their actions on social networks. As such, this shifts the role of media in identity construction toward an even more dynamic ecology. In particular, it raises questions regarding children's privacy and social media's interest of maximizing data collection for marketing purpose.

Second, adolescents' use of social media bridges both virtual and physical space. Since many social networks require that users register with their real names, effective segmentation of online and offline conduct becomes functionally impossible. Further, adolescents' conduct online is increasingly paired with their conduct offline and used, for example, by colleges and future employers to screen candidates[2]. In traditional media contexts, by contrast, an adolescents' content consumption,

---

[1] Amanda Lenhart, Kristen Purcell, Aaron Smith, Kathryn Zickuhr, Social Media and Young Adults, Feb 3, 2010, http://www.pewinternet.org/Reports/2010/Social-Media-and-Young-Adults.aspx.

[2] According to some studies, as high as 90% of employers screen candidates by looking at social media profiles. See, e.g., Lindsay Olson, Employers Will Check Your Social Media Profiles, US News, October 27, 2011, http://money.usnews.com/money/blogs/outside-voices-careers/2011/10/27/employers-will-check-your-social-media-profiles.

though impacting her development, is not generally used as a screening mechanism for important educational and occupational opportunities years later. Gone is the 'safe space' of adolescent identity experimentation that many adolescents have relied on in order to grow.

Third, social media not only intermediates content but – more importantly – it intermediates the creation of identity. In the words of Eric Schmidt, Google's former CEO, a social network such as Google+ isn't just a website, it's an 'identity service'[3]. Instead of simply providing content *to* users in internet spaces, social networks now also provide information *about* users. Stated another way, harms are possible to adolescents not only from visible content on social networks, but also from the invisible privacy-invasive acts of intermediaries behind the scenes. Intermediaries, such as social networks, frequently act in part as information aggregators, selling profiles of their users based on user's interests, demographics and internet histories[4]. Through this data aggregation and profiling, intermediaries begin to construct a story about the adolescent, frequently driven by demographic generalizations, which may include racial stereotypes. An adolescent's self-constructed identity increasingly may be at odds with the identity that Google or Facebook chooses to construct for her (and share with third parties).

Intermediaries, such as social networks, increasingly usurp the power to manage users' identities away from users. The user's desired salient role identity may become overshadowed by the identity that the intermediary instead chooses to project for that user. Intermediaries, particularly social media, are built by design to push users into a highly integrated identity hierarchy; usually, the intermediary chooses to integrate all known role identities for a user – both online and offline – regardless of the user's salience hierarchy or preferences. In essence, the choice of a segmented role identity becomes almost impossible in a highly intermediated world of information. As a consequence, the types of harms implicated by media today have evolved to include these new types of privacy and identity building harms that are worthy of further exploration in future work.

[3] Matt Rosoff, Google+ Isn't Just A Social Network, It's An "Identity Service", Business Insider, Aug. 28, 2011, http://www.businessinsider.com/google-isnt-just-a-social-network-its-an-identity-service-2011–8.

[4] Meanwhile, the user may not be aware that these particular third parties have access to her clickstream and other data. According to some studies, as high as 90% of employers screen candidates by looking at social media profiles. See, e.g., Lindsay Olson, Employers Will Check Your Social Media Profiles, US News, October 27, 2011, http://money.usnews.com/money/blogs/outside-voices-careers/2011/10/27/employers-will-check-your-social-media-profiles.

Andrea M. Matwyshyn
University of Pennsylvania
3700 Walnut Street
Philadelphia, PA 19104–6216 (USA)
E-Mail amatwysh@wharton.upenn.edu

Dr. Andrea Matwyshyn (PhD 2005 in the Program on Human Development and Social Policy; JD, Northwestern University 1999 in the School of Law) is Assistant Professor of Legal Studies and Business Ethics at the Wharton School, University of Pennsylvania, and has been an Affiliate, at the Centre for Economics and Policy at the University of Cambridge since 2003. She specializes in internet technology regulation and corporate law. In 2009, Stanford University Press published her edited volume: *Harboring data, information security, law and the corporation*.

Slaughter-Defoe DT (ed): Racial Stereotyping and Child Development.
Contrib Hum Dev. Basel, Karger, 2012, vol 25, pp 57–79

'What Does Race Have to Do with Math?' Relationships between Racial-Mathematical Socialization, Mathematical Identity, and Racial Identity

Traci L. English-Clarke[a] · Diana T. Slaughter-Defoe[a] · Danny B. Martin[b]

[a]University of Pennsylvania, Philadelphia, Pa., and [b]University of Illinois, Chicago, Ill., USA

Abstract

In this chapter, we focus on the racial-mathematical socialization stories and messages reported by African-American youth and the significance of these stories and messages in terms of youths' mathematical identities. We also examine the relationship between racial-mathematical beliefs and youths' mathematical and racial identities. In examining youths' negotiation of racial-mathematical stereotypes, we found that racial identity constructs were more closely related to racial-mathematical beliefs for 10th graders than for 9th graders. This suggests that as youths' racial identities develop, their understandings about race increasingly affect their racial-mathematical beliefs. Additionally, about one-third of the interviewed youth reported hearing racial-mathematical messages or stories from parents or other people. The majority of these stories and messages described racial discrimination in a mathematical setting, while others touched on racial-mathematical stereotypes or the dearth of African-Americans in high-level mathematics. Racial-mathematical socialization may serve as a special support for youth rather than just an additional context for racial socialization; youth who hear racial-mathematical socialization stories or messages may develop a deeper and more complex understanding of the far-reaching effects of discrimination, the youth-relevant contexts in which discrimination can occur, and the racial imbalances that they may perceive and experience as they reach higher levels of mathematics.

Copyright © 2012 S. Karger AG, Basel

One's personal identity has been theorized to develop over time and in response to one's experiences, including environment-based risks, protective factors, situation-based challenges, and supports that protect against these challenges [Spencer, 1995]. Socialization messages, including racial socialization, can serve as a challenge or support for youth, depending on the content of the socialization messages and the ways in which

Author note: This chapter stems from the first author's dissertation research, which focused on mathematical, racial, and racial-mathematical socialization messages and stories and their role in shaping African-American youths' mathematical identities. In the dissertation, mixed methods were used to explore the relationships between racial and mathematical socialization and identity by analyzing surveys of 263 youth of various races (168 African-American) in 9th and 10th grades and in-depth, one-on-one interviews with 28 African-American youth. English-Clarke examined the mathematical, racial, and racial-mathematical socialization received by African-American youth, as well as the ways in which the youth perceived and used this socialization.

the youth perceive them. Mathematical identity for African-American youth is likely similar to personal identity in that it develops over time and in response to an individual's experiences [Berry, 2008; Jackson, 2009; McGee, 2009; Martin, 2000, 2006, 2007, 2009; McGee & Martin, 2011; Spencer, 2009; Stinson, 2006, 2009, 2011]. However, for African-Americans, the experiences influencing mathematical identity not only include classroom-based and out-of-school mathematical experiences, but also socialization stories or messages from parents and the larger society involving both race and mathematics. For example, some African-American adults and parents feel a need to help African-American children overcome negative thinking that mathematics is for others and that mathematics participation is determined by race [Martin, 2000, 2006, 2007].

This chapter will examine the linkages between race and mathematics from the perspectives of African-American youth. First, we explore racial-mathematical socialization stories and messages reported by African-American youth and the significance of these stories and messages in terms of youths' mathematical identities. We then investigate youths' racial-mathematical beliefs (primarily racial stereotypes about math). We also examine the relationship between racial-mathematical beliefs and youths' mathematical and racial identities.

Background

Theoretical Framework
Educational research and interventions based on models of psychosocial and cognitive development that take for granted European and European American, middle-class norms may not be relevant to the lives of youth from other cultures, and thus may not bring about the researchers' desired understanding [Gordon, 1990; Lee, Spencer & Harpalani, 2003; Tillman, 2002]. For many years, theorists tended to view youths' motivation to achieve in school as largely irrelevant of social,

cultural, and environmental context – neither social position variables nor experiences of racism and segregation are explicitly examined in these models [i.e., Dweck, 1999; Eccles, 1997; Nicholls, 1984; Wigfield & Eccles, 2000]. Mathematics education researchers as well as those examining Black-White achievement differences also tended to ignore the social conditions and realities of those populations they were studying, or viewed negative outcomes for African-Americans as a result of cultural deficits [Slaughter-Defoe, 1995]. However, there has been a push in recent years to investigate the social contexts in which individuals live – including issues around social class, race/ethnicity, culture, language, gender, sexuality, and more – and to include their daily life experiences as a factor in their life processes and outcomes [Nasir & Saxe, 2003; Oyserman, Gant & Ager, 1995; Spencer, 1995; Spencer et al., 2006].

Spencer's Phenomenological Variant of Ecological Systems Theory (PVEST) helps to elucidate some of these contextual components and variables and the ways in which they might interact with daily experiences to form a youth's identity over time [Spencer, 1995]. PVEST (fig. 1) is a framework that is designed to help us understand the normative development of people belonging to different racial and ethnic groups, social classes, and genders.

It invites us to look closely at the individual risks and protective factors in an individual's or group's environment, along with the challenges one faces and the supports that protect against these challenges. The framework includes the coping strategies that individuals use to deal with their net stress level (challenges and supports combined), allowing us to categorize the strategies as adaptive or maladaptive according to the immediate outcomes in a given context. The framework also includes the emergent identities, the positive and negative stable coping responses that are developed when the coping strategies are used over time, and the coping outcomes (productive or unproductive) that result. This is a recursive model,

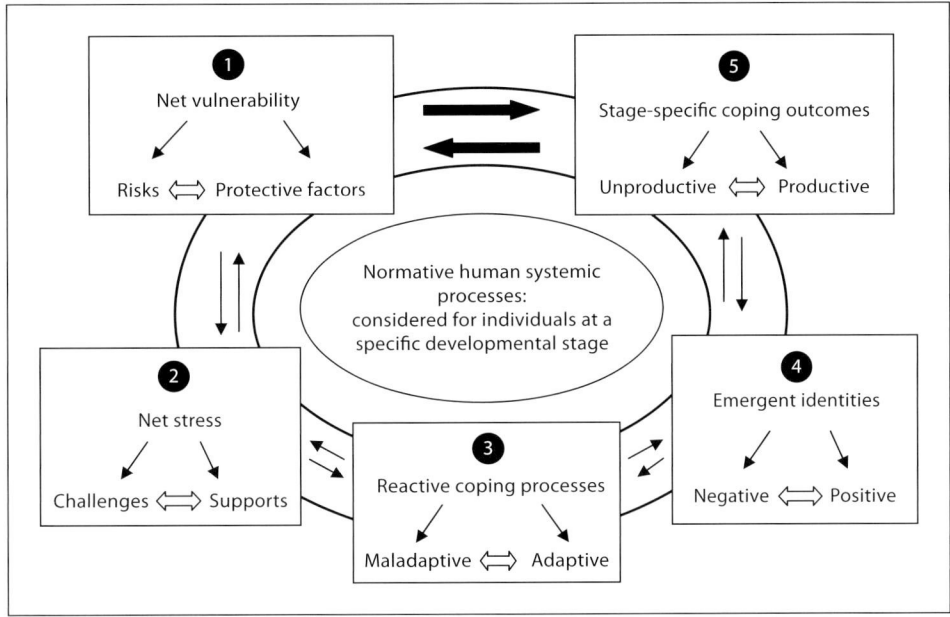

Fig. 1. Phenomenological Variant of Ecological Systems Theory (PVEST). Spencer et al. [2006, p. 641], reprinted with permission.

in that outcomes at one point in time can become risk or protective factors, or even challenges or supports, later on in the individual's experience.

This framework is helpful in that it allows us to dig deeper into the meanings that African-American adolescents construct, as well as the behaviors that they exhibit, towards math in school based on their experiences and socialization around race and mathematics. Youth are not empty vessels when they arrive at school each day – they experience socialization around race and mathematics that influences how they respond to mathematics in their classrooms. Learning about this socialization and the ways in which African-American youth negotiate the messages that they receive – be they explicit or implicit, verbal or nonverbal – will allow us to better understand their coping strategies and the processes that lead to youths' racial and mathematical identities.

Next, we briefly discuss identity development for youth, especially as it pertains to their racial identity development. As African-American youths' identities around mathematics may be related to their identities around race [Berry, 2008; Martin, 2000], we must examine theories about adolescent identity in general and racial identity in particular before we can begin to understand mathematical identity for this group of youth.

Identity Development
During adolescence, youth begin to question various aspects of their identities such as belief systems, social structures, personal values, and roles. For the purposes of this chapter, we use a definition of identity in the Eriksonian tradition, 'an ongoing dynamic process whereby individuals establish, evaluate, reevaluate, and reestablish who they are and are not relative to others in their environments' [Chatman, Eccles & Malanchuk, 2005, p. 117]. Erik Erikson's theory of identity development states that adolescents experience an identity crisis that is most pronounced during this life

stage. This identity crisis is never fully resolved, as identity issues are frequently reevaluated in the face of major life changes. During this initial identity crisis, however, the adolescent is faced with the task of establishing 'a sense of personal identity' and avoiding the dangers of 'role diffusion' and 'identity confusion', which could lead to self-destructive behaviors. The adolescent must resolve issues regarding who she/he is, where she/he came from, and who she/he wants to become. In other words, identity construction involves establishing a meaningful self-concept that brings together one's past, present, and future. When adolescents begin to construct and negotiate their identities, they tend to seek feedback from older generations, peers, and others, as the various aspects of identity can only be found through interaction with significant others. During this process, there is a preoccupation with how one appears in the eyes of others, in order to compare this perception to how one feels and strives to be. Eventually, the adolescent achieves a mature identity, which gives her/him a sense of knowing where she/he is headed and a self-assurance that she/he will receive recognition from those who matter the most [Muuss, 1996].

Building on Erikson's theory, James Marcia further hypothesized that adolescents' identity development consists of four non-hierarchical phases: identity-diffused, foreclosure, moratorium, and identity-achieved. The identity-diffused youth has not yet had an identity crisis and has not explored various roles or beliefs, nor has she/he personally committed to particular goals, values, or beliefs. The youth in the status of foreclosure has not yet had an identity crisis, but she/he has made a commitment to certain goals, values, and beliefs based solely on socialization by parents or significant others. The moratorium status is one in which the adolescent is in a state of exploration, and thus tries on many different roles or values in search of the ones that suit her or him, but has not yet made a permanent commitment to any in particular. The identity-achieved status is one of

completion, in which the youth has resolved his or her identity issues through exploration. She/he has made a well-defined personal commitment to particular beliefs, roles, and values. Being in a certain identity status can have implications for one's self-concept, level of anxiety, and other aspects of emotional experience [Muuss, 1996].

Racial Identity Development
The exploration of one's racial identity may not be an important issue for majority-race adolescents, as it is not necessarily a salient aspect of their personal identity [Phinney & Alipuria, 1990; Rotheram-Borus, 1989, as cited in Muuss, 1996]. However, together with general identity search issues, adolescents who are members of racial minority groups may also begin to actively search for racial identities [Spencer & Markstrom-Adams, 1990]. For African-Americans, 'Blackness' is said to perform three functions in everyday African-American life: defending the individual from the negative psychological stress of living in a racist society; providing a sense of purpose, affiliation and meaning, and providing psychological mechanisms that facilitate social interaction with non-African-American people, situations and cultures [Cross, 1991]. It is likely that other racial identities perform similar functions (specific to the group) which seem essential for life in a society where many individuals have different racial and cultural experiences from one's own.

Most researchers hold the theoretical perspective that the process of racial identity development is similar to that of Erikson and Marcia's model for other aspects of identity development, in that there are four general phases: (1) Initially, youth have the attitudes of those around them, and (2) at some point they encounter a situation or series of events that cause them to question their racial identity and the role of race in their world. They then go through two other phases during which they (3) try on other attitudes and challenge those around them, and (4) finally settle on an identity that works for them [Bennett, 2006; Phinney

& Chavira, 1995; Phinney & Ong, 2007; Seaton, Scottham & Sellers, 2006].

Research on ethnic and racial identity development suggests that African-American youth, as well as other minority youth, may have many identity tasks to accomplish during adolescence that reach far beyond the identity tasks of Caucasian American youth. Researchers such as Helms [2007] have developed theories that detail the racial identity development of Whites, but they suggest that White racial identity development often occurs at a much later age than for minority youth [Tatum, 1997]. Exploring one's racial identity is simply more salient for African-Americans than for White youth, although members of both races may have begun to think about and search for a racial identity by the 8th grade [Rotheram-Borus, 1989, as cited in Muuss, 1996]. The main reason for this greater salience is that African-American youth and other minority youth realize at a young age that they are seen as members of a group rather than as individuals [Tatum, 1997]. They realize that they are not like those around them – in fact, that they are living in a society in which most of the people portrayed in the media, government, positions of power, and people who are considered to embody universal standards of beauty do not look or sound anything like them. Additionally, these youth usually face discrimination and racism in their daily lives, or at the very least, they hear about racism from their parents and other adults around them. Caucasian youth growing up in mostly White neighborhoods tend to consider themselves to be racially 'normal' – they see race largely as belonging to minorities [Tatum, 1997]. They typically do not experience racism and thus do not tend to think about their race as a major factor in their identities.

Content of a Racial Identity

Phinney and Ong [2007] reviewed several components of racial and ethnic identity content that have been explored with adolescent populations: self-categorization and labeling, commitment and attachment, exploration, behavioral involvement, in-group attitudes or private regard, ethnic values and beliefs, importance or salience of group membership, and ethnic identity in relation to national identity. Self-categorization is simply identifying oneself as a member of a particular social group, and is a basic element of ethnic/racial identity. Commitment refers to one's attachment to and personal investment in a group. These researchers suggest that commitment is the most important aspect of racial/ethnic identity. Commitment is one major aspect of Marcia's expansion of Erikson's theory for adolescent identity [Muuss, 1996]; along with exploration, it determines an individual's location in the phases of the status model. Exploration is the search for experiences and information that are relevant to one's developing identity. Without exploration, one's commitment to a particular identity is likely somewhat tenuous. Evaluation and in-group attitudes consist of one's attitudes about one's own racial group. This is sometimes referred to as private regard [Sellers et al., 1997; Scottham, Sellers & Nguyen, 2008].

Because of the social and cultural history of African-Americans, many cultural practices and beliefs were formed in opposition to and/or in order to cope with racism, discrimination, and societal racial socialization [Slaughter-Defoe, Johnson & Spencer, 2009]. As a result, the socially constructed concept of race has had a very real impact on the experiences of African-Americans [Sellers et al., 1998]. While it is potentially feasible to separate some African-American cultural practices from the impact of racism and racial dynamics on the individual, the two are not fully mutually exclusive. For instance, watching Black TV shows and going to Black movies could be considered both an effort to support Black entertainment (an impact of racism and racial dynamics) and an act of participation in the cultural practices of African-Americans.

Sellers and his colleagues define racial identity for African-Americans as 'the significance and qualitative meaning that individuals attribute to their membership within the Black racial group within their self-concepts' [Sellers et al., 1998, p. 23]. Thus, for their model, the Multidimensional Model of Racial Identity (MMRI), racial identity consists of the importance that an individual places on race in his/her self-perceptions as well as the individual's conception of what it means to be Black. The MMRI is a multidimensional model of African-American identity that incorporates four dimensions: (1) Ideology, or one's beliefs about what it means to be Black and ways Black people should behave, (2) Centrality, the degree to which race and racial identity are normally central to one's overall identity, (3) Regard, the ways in which the individual views Blacks and the ways in which the individual perceives that others view Blacks, and (4) Salience, the degree to which race is a relevant aspect of one's self-concept at a given moment in time [Sellers et al., 1997, 1998]. This model uses a phenomenological approach to studying racial identity; that is, a focus on the individual's perception of his/her experiences and identity. The MMRI is concerned mainly with the status and nature of the racial identity versus its development. This differentiates it from other, earlier models of racial identity (e.g. Cross; Phinney) that are focused primarily on identity development; however, it is not theoretically incompatible with those models, but complementary [Sellers et al., 1998].

Outcomes Related to Racial Identity

African-American and other minority college students who had explored and successfully established a commitment to a racial identity had significantly higher self-esteem than those who had not [Seaton, Scottham & Sellers, 2006]. Simply searching for a racial identity was also found to be related to self-esteem for African-American and Mexican-American students [Phinney & Alipuria, 1990]. Likewise, individuals who were diffused with regard to racial identity reported more depressive symptoms than those who were

in a moratorium or foreclosed stage, who in turn reported more depressive symptoms than those who had an achieved racial identity [Yip, Seaton & Sellers, 2006]. Findings such as these suggest that the search for and achievement of a racial identity is an extremely important part of identity development for African American adolescents, and is one of the many issues they must contend with in the midst of schooling. As such, racial identity may be connected to other aspects of identity for African-American youth, such as their identities around mathematics.

Before an individual encounters an event or situation that causes a questioning of racial identity, he or she has already become enculturated into a racial group by his or her parents, family members, and broader community. This takes place through racial socialization, which is discussed in the next section. Racial socialization occurs continuously throughout one's life; it does not start only when an individual begins to actively search for a racial identity, nor does it cease when she/he has achieved a fairly stable racial identity.

Racial Socialization

For many families with racial background(s) that are considered a minority in the United States, and thus are culturally, physically, and historically different from the mainstream, a central component of parenting involves communicating with children about race and its potential impact on and importance in the child's life. Racial socialization has been defined as 'the mechanisms through which parents transmit information, values, and perspectives about . . . race to their children' [Hughes et al., 2006, p. 747]. This includes mechanisms that allow children to negotiate the contexts in which they live, which in the United States today may contain high levels of racial, ethnic, and cultural diversity [Hughes et al., 2006]. Parents or other adults may talk with the child about the differences they see and experiences they may have, cook foods or play types of music that are central to their culture, decorate their homes with culture-specific artwork or decorations, or even involve the child in classes or groups that teach culture-specific language, music, religion, or dance. This type of socialization is meant to help the child to coexist with people who are different than him or her, to value the home culture, to live with the racism he or she may encounter, and/or to allow him or her to deal with difference and discrimination effectively on a daily basis and in the long-term. Racial socialization is considered a protective factor in the lives of youth [Hughes & Chen, 1997; Neblett et al., 2008], and for African-American populations, it has been found to serve as a buffer against racial discrimination experiences [Bynum, Burton & Best, 2007]. Racial socialization can take the form of direct or indirect messages, verbal or nonverbal modes, and overt or covert styles. Family members may be unaware of some of the socialization practices in their family, such as their actions, interactions, and reactions in everyday life, both inside and outside of their home and community. Most of the research on racial socialization focuses on overt socialization practices, such as messages or verbal directives given to children; less common is for research to measure modeled behaviors, opportunities provided, and interactive experiences [Brown, Linver, Evans & DeGennaro, 2009; Brown, Linver & Evans, 2010].

Components of Racial Socialization

Hughes et al. [2006] conducted a meta-analysis of 45 research studies on racial socialization, and identified a lack of standardized terminology and measurement, which causes difficulty for summarizing findings across the field. They proposed four main category labels to represent the major types of socialization content identified in the studies: (a) preparation for bias, (b) cultural socialization, (c) egalitarianism, and (d) promotion of mistrust. Preparation for bias is a term that describes parents' attempts to inform their children about racial barriers and create an awareness of discrimination, as well as to prepare the children

to cope with these problems. Cultural socialization describes parents' attempts to provide their children with knowledge and pride about the history, traditions, and culture of their racial group. Egalitarianism describes parents' efforts to emphasize to children the value of hard work and developing skills that will help them to succeed in mainstream culture settings. These parents emphasize individual characteristics over cultural membership. Promotion of mistrust refers to parents' efforts to emphasize the need for caution and distrust around people of other races. These efforts typically do not include strategies for interacting with people of other races, except perhaps implying that one should keep one's distance, emotionally or physically.

Certain combinations of racial socialization message types have been found to have the most positive outcomes for children, both academically and psychologically [Stevenson, Cameron, Herrero-Taylor & Davis, 2002]. This suggests that there is an optimal balance of types of racial socialization, and that not all racial socialization necessarily has a positive impact on children. As a result, the array of racial socialization that some children experience may serve as a protective factor or a support, while the array of racial socialization that other children experience may serve as a risk factor or a challenge, doing the child more harm than good. Parents may not be aware of the potentially positive or negative impact of certain types of socialization, the amount of socialization occurring, or of their focus on one theme to the detriment of another [Brown, Linver, Evans & DeGennaro, 2009; Neblett et al., 2008].

While the racial socialization literature focuses on socialization messages that are disconnected from specific academic disciplines, we have found that some youth also experience racial socialization that is related to the discipline of mathematics [Berry, 2008; McGee, 2010; Martin, 2000, 2006, 2007; McGee & Martin, 2011; Stinson, 2006, 2009]. We call this *racial-mathematical socialization*. Berry [2008] provides an example of this socialization with a student named Cordell, who explains that his mother communicated to him that she believed he faced racial discrimination in his school math course placement. 'The teacher and principal did not want me tested [for the gifted math program] because they felt I was not gifted. My mother thinks the reason they did not want to test me was because I am Black. She stayed on the teachers and principals until I was tested. I did well enough to be placed in the [academically gifted] program midway through my 4th-grade year'. This newly uncovered type of socialization has not been overtly examined by research studies; thus, there is little literature on this aspect of socialization. Racial-mathematical socialization is likely related to African-American youths' views of math as well as to their performance in math, especially since racial socialization seems to be closely related to academic outcomes.

Mathematical Socialization

In addition to experiencing socialization about race, African-American youth (along with youth of other races) experience socialization about mathematics that is not implicitly or explicitly connected to issues of race. As with racial-mathematical socialization, mathematical socialization has not been studied extensively, but is likely to consist of both socialization about what it means to do mathematics and socialization for success or failure in mathematics. Martin [2007, p. 8] conceptualized mathematics socialization as 'the experiences that individuals and groups have within a variety of contexts such as school, family, peer groups, and the workplace that legitimize or inhibit meaningful participation in mathematics'. Similar to Hughes et al.'s [2006, p. 747] definition of racial socialization, 'the mechanisms through which parents transmit information, values, and perspectives about ethnicity and race to their children', we assert that through the mechanisms of mathematical socialization, parents transmit information, values, and perspectives about mathematics and participation in mathematics to their children.

Since African-American adults in the 1950s, 1960s, and 1970s were often tracked out of higher-level mathematics courses in school or were dissuaded from majoring in mathematics and the sciences primarily because of their race, mathematics seems to have a racialized character in African-American communities [Martin, 2000, 2006, 2007]. In his interviews with African-American parents about their experiences with mathematics, Martin found that parents brought up the ways in which racism affected their view of mathematics and their trajectory in math throughout their schooling. Depending on the parents' internalization of these experiences, their socialization of their children seemed to place them into one of two categories: (1) parents who insisted that their children do well in math (sometimes even helping the child with math homework) and strongly advocated for their child when they perceived racial discrimination affecting their child's placement or grades, and (2) parents who did not expect their child to do very well in math and did not push them to do better than 'just passing'. The latter parents had a negative view about mathematics, while the former parents had a positive view of math, despite all having similar experiences with math-related racial discrimination as youth [Martin, 2000]. These findings suggest that parents' take on their mathematical experiences, and their view of the racism they may have encountered in the pursuit of mathematical knowledge, impact youths' views of and behaviors toward mathematics.

Mathematical Identity

Mathematical identity is distinct from mathematics self-concept and self-efficacy in that these constructs are typically operationalized as task-based and situational, whereas we conceive of mathematical identity to be a more stable and overarching construct that is achieved through a process similar to identity development for other domains and can change over time based on a person's experiences and perceptions. Through the lens of the PVEST framework, mathematical identity could be viewed as an emergent identity that develops over time, formed from one's risks (such as being female or having learning difficulties specific to mathematics), protective factors (such as a mathematically enriched environment), challenges (such as discrimination in math-related settings or negative interactions with teachers around math) and supports (such as access to math tutors or teachers who believe in one's capability), and maladaptive/adaptive reactive coping strategies (such as high or low mathematical self-concept or self-efficacy, mathematical persistence or lack thereof, help-seeking, viewing math as useless, etc.). As with racial identity and identities in other domains, the salience of one's mathematical identity may vary situationally, and may change over time if the individual has an experience that causes him/her to question or re-explore his or her mathematical identity.

Youths' attitudes about math are closely related to their mathematical identities, and are a reasonable, though incomplete, approximation of their mathematical identities at any given time. Four major components of math attitudes are generally examined, and are based on revisions of the Fennema and Sherman [1976] measure of math attitudes: confidence, effectance motivation, perceived usefulness of math, and perceived maleness of math. Confidence is typically defined as one's confidence in their mathematical abilities overall. Effectance motivation is often described as interest in math, but Fennema and Sherman's measures seem to actualize it as a combination of the degree to which one shows active involvement in mathematics and the degree to which one enjoys, seeks out, and persists at challenging mathematical tasks. Perceived usefulness of math is the degree to which youth perceive mathematics as useful for their lives, and maleness is the degree to which one perceives of math as a male-oriented domain.

All of these constructs play a part in youths' mathematical identities, along with one's history of experiences with mathematics. Because identities in different domains may be related to each other, it is possible that African-American youths' mathematical identities are linked to their racial identities. Specifically, if youth perceived their experiences with mathematics to be related somehow to race or to racial discrimination, their mathematical identities and racial identities may be interconnected as a result.

Racial-Mathematical Identity
Martin's work [1997, 2000, 2006, 2007] highlights possible linkages between African-American mathematical identity and racial identity. He defines mathematics identity as 'the dispositions and deeply held beliefs that individuals develop about their ability to participate and perform effectively in mathematical contexts and to use mathematics to change the conditions of their lives' [Martin, 2007, pp. 8–9]. Mathematics identity also involves one's understandings about how they see themselves and are seen by others in mathematical contexts.

Martin argues that for African-Americans, racial identity is inextricable from mathematical identity [2007]. From his interviews with African-American parents and adults, he has found that many African-Americans who were educated in the 1950s, 1960s, and 1970s experienced mathematics learning and participation as racialized – they felt that they were viewed or treated negatively in the realm of learning mathematics, primarily due to their race. Many of these adults felt a 'need to expose African-American children to role models in mathematics to overcome negative thinking that mathematics is for others and that who does and does not do mathematics is determined by race' [Martin, 2006, p. 202]. Thus, it seems that adults with these types of experiences might consciously or unconsciously socialize their children with regard to their experiences, beliefs, and values about mathematics as they relate to race, i.e. racial-mathematical socialization.

Research Questions

Unfortunately, racial-mathematical socialization has not been studied extensively, either in the form of socialization about race that is related to the field of mathematics, or in the form of socialization about mathematics that has a racial component. This is an area that could contribute to our understanding of African-American youths' performance in mathematics, and thus to addressing the dearth of African-Americans in fields that require advanced mathematical knowledge. Additionally, understanding racial-mathematical socialization and its relationship to African-American youths' racial and mathematical identities could assist teachers and parents in reducing the racial achievement gap in mathematics.

In this research, the primary author explored the following questions: (a) What types of racial-mathematical socialization messages and stories are passed along to African-American youth, and how do youth respond to these socialization messages/stories? What significance do these stories have in terms of youths' mathematical identities? (b) Do most African-American youth share certain racial-mathematical beliefs, and are these beliefs related to gender or grades in math? (c) How are racial-mathematical beliefs related to mathematical identity and racial identity for African-American youth?

Method

Procedure

One hundred and sixty-eight 9th and 10th grade Black or African-American youth were surveyed to elicit their attitudes towards mathematics, the ways in which they have been socialized around race and around mathematics, elements of their racial identities, and messages they have received about mathematics and about race. Surveys took approximately 20 min to complete, and were available in both paper and electronic versions; a few sample items are provided below. The questions on both versions of the survey were identical, except that for a few questions (such as grade level and typical math grades), the

online version allowed participants to select only one response, and the online version also required a response for a few key questions (such as grade level and race/ethnicity). Students were not compensated for their participation in the survey.

The students were chosen from three high schools in the metropolitan area of a Northeastern city. Galena school was a medium-sized magnet public school with sizeable populations of African-American, Caucasian, Latino, and Asian students, Obsidian school was a small, mostly-African-American charter school whose students lived in various parts of the city, and Azurite school was a large, mostly White suburban public school with a sizeable African-American student population and a small Asian-American population; this school's students came from the upper-middle class neighborhood in which it was located. All three schools had good academic reputations, but Obsidian students generally scored much lower on standardized tests than students at the other two schools, and at Azurite, African-American students generally scored far below students of other races on standardized tests. The sample consisted of 44.0% male students (74), 55.4% female students (93), and 0.6% transgender students (1). All youth in this sample self-identified as Black or African-American, including several youth who were racially mixed as well as a few youth with Afro-Caribbean or African parentage. The sample was fairly diverse socioeconomically, as measured by mother's educational attainment; 30.4% of youth reported that their mother had a high school diploma or less, 27.3% reported that their mother had some post-secondary education, and 42.4% reported that their mother had attained at least a 4-year college degree.

Twenty-eight of the youth surveyed were later interviewed about the socialization they received from parents and others regarding mathematics and race, focusing on overt stories or messages that were passed along to them. Interviews with students generally took place during students' lunch periods in an empty classroom at their school. These interviews typically took about 35–45 min each, although a few interviews lasted longer than an hour. At the conclusion of the interview, students were given USD 10 in appreciation for their time. Youth were specifically asked whether they had ever heard a message or story about someone's experiences with math that had to do with race, as well as about messages or stories about someone's experiences with race or racism that had to do with math. We will refer to these messages and stories as *racial-mathematical messages and stories*. Students were also asked about their reactions to the stories and messages they had heard. The interviewed youth included nine males, one transgender student, and 18 females. Two youths specified that they were Jamaican American. When the interview participants began their participation in the study, 11 were 9th graders and 17 were 10th graders.

Measures
Racial-Mathematical Attitudes
Measures of racial-mathematical attitudes were developed for this study, and were assessed through the *Youth Survey on Race and Mathematics* [English-Clarke, 2011]. This 38-item measure consists of five subscales, and was designed to elicit teenagers': (1) attitudes about math, (2) experiences with math and race, (3) knowledge of parents' and others' experiences with math, (4) knowledge of parents' and others' experiences with school, and (5) racial-mathematical stereotypes and beliefs. This questionnaire consists predominately of closed-ended questions, which were posed as statements with which participants were asked to rate their agreement on a 5-point Likert-type scale ranging from strongly agree to strongly disagree.

The seven-item subscale on racial-mathematical stereotypes and beliefs is designed to assess students' level of agreement with various stereotypes and beliefs that address both math and race. This subscale consists of four mini-subscales, each addressing a different type of racial-mathematical belief: (1) Black racial math performance beliefs, (2) Black math student performance beliefs, (3) math discrimination beliefs, and (4) Asian-American math performance beliefs. Two sample items from this subscale are: 'Asian-Americans are better in math than people of other races' and 'The popular Black students in my school don't do well in math'.

Math Attitudes
Attitudes about math were assessed by a subscale on the *Youth Survey on Race and Mathematics (YSRM)*. This subscale consists of nine questions, eight of which were derived from the *Revised Math Attitude Survey (RMAS)* [P.T. Reid & S.K. Roberts, pers. commun., April 1, 2005], a revision of the Fennema-Sherman Mathematics Attitudes Scales. The 50-item *RMAS* has 4 subscales, designed to assess: (1) confidence in the subject matter of math, (2) perceived usefulness of math content, (3) perception of math as a male domain[1], and (4) effectance motivation, which ranges from lack of involvement in mathematics to active enjoyment of and seeking challenge in math as a subject matter [Fennema & Sherman, 1976]. Questions were posed as statements, and students were asked to rate their agreement with each statement on a 5-point Likert scale ranging from 'strongly agree' to 'strongly disagree', with 'not sure' as the midpoint. Items were coded so that a higher value was assigned to greater endorsement of the construct. For the math attitude subscale on the *YSRM*, questions were taken from all four of the subscales from the *RMAS*, with two questions each from the confidence, usefulness, and effectance motivation subscales and one question from the perception of math as a male domain

subscale[2]. The *YSRM* math attitude subscale also includes a question on the perceived usefulness of math that was taken from a longer version of the *RMAS*.

Racial Identity
To assess youth racial identity, students completed the *Multidimensional Inventory of Black Identity-Teen* [Scottham et al., 2008]. This 21-item measure consists of four subscales and is designed to assess various aspects of Black teenagers' racial identity. It is based on the constructs in the adult-centered Multidimensional Inventory of Black Identity (MIBI), and was developed specifically for use with adolescents. The Centrality subscale measures the extent to which the individual feels that race is an important aspect of his/her identity. A higher score on this subscale indicates that race is a more central part of one's identity. The Private Regard subscale measures how positive the individual feels about other African-Americans and about being African-American. On this subscale, a higher score indicates more positive feelings about African-Americans. The Public Regard subscale measures the individual's perception of other groups' feelings towards African-Americans. A higher score on this subscale reflects a more positive perception of others' views towards African-Americans. The Ideology subscale is divided into four subscales, each indicating how the individual feels that African-Americans should act. Higher scores on each of these subscales indicate endorsement of that ideology. The ideology subscales are: (a) Assimilationist, (b) Humanist, (c) Oppressed Minority, and (d) Nationalist. Assimilationist ideology is an orientation towards assimilating with the mainstream European American culture, both ideologically and geographically, whereas Humanist ideology is an orientation towards emphasizing the importance of being an individual over being a member of a particular racial group. Oppressed Minority ideology is an orientation towards emphasizing the similarities among all oppressed minority groups, including African-Americans, and Nationalist ideology is an orientation towards emphasizing and supporting the distinctive value of African-American culture, history, and society.

Student Characteristics
Students' demographic characteristics were assessed by measures on the *YSRM* which included questions about race, gender, ethnic background, grade level in school, mother's educational attainment (as a proxy for

---

[1] Maleness was not used in any of the analyses presented here.

[2] Questions from the RMAS were repeated on the YSRM because while all participants were to complete the YSRM, only about a third of participants were scheduled to complete the RMAS. The repeated questions allowed the researcher to gather some information about the math attitudes of those students not completing the RMAS and to thereby include all participants in analyses of math attitudes.

socioeconomic status), student's desired educational attainment, average grades in school, and average grades in mathematics.

Survey Distribution

Each student who participated in the survey was given two questionnaires. All students first received the *Youth Survey on Race and Mathematics* (*YSRM*), and students also completed one of the following three questionnaires:

- Revised Math Attitude Survey (RMAS)
- Teenager Experience of Racial Socialization (TERS)[3]
- Multidimensional Inventory of Black Identity-Teen (MIBI-T)

Youth were assigned to complete one of these three questionnaires in order to minimize the time needed for each student to complete the survey, as well as to ensure that relatively equal numbers of African-American students would complete each of these questionnaires. African-American students were randomly assigned to complete the second questionnaire to eliminate bias in assigning the questionnaires to students. No known characteristic was associated with receiving a particular questionnaire[4].

Findings

Racial-Mathematical Stories and Messages

About a third of interviewed youth reported hearing a story or message from their parents or other adults (i.e., teachers, family members, and friends), that involved both math and race. While most of these youth reported only hearing one such message or story, one girl reported having heard two racial-mathematical messages or stories. The relative infrequency of these reported messages is striking given the ubiquity of race in society as well as the 'racial achievement gap', which is often publicly discussed in urban schools. Messages and stories that involved both math and race fell into three main categories: (1) stories or messages about racism and racial discrimination in a math setting, (2) stories or messages about persistence despite being one of few Blacks in a math class, and (3) messages about Asians' performance in math.

About 45% of the messages and stories focused on racial discrimination or racism in math settings; this discrimination was often perpetrated by students or individual teachers rather than being primarily structural or institution-based. Approximately 18% of the messages or stories focused on persisting despite being one of few Black students in a math class, and about 27% of the racial-mathematical messages conveyed that Asian Americans performed highly in mathematics. While the other types of racial-mathematical socialization messages/stories were typically transmitted by parents or other adults, messages about Asians' high performance in math were typically transmitted by friends or other students.

Below are some examples of each type of racial-mathematical socialization messages and stories provided by youth interviewed for this study, along with the youths' reactions to these messages and stories.

Persisting Despite Few African-Americans in Math Classes

Benjamin, a 10th grade student at Azurite school, indicated that his parents warned him that there would be very few African-Americans as he got into higher-level math classes. At the time of the interview, Benjamin had recently begun 11th grade and was one of the two African-American students at his school taking B.C. Calculus, the highest level A.P. Calculus class available.

Benjamin: I don't think they've told me any stories, but they've said how the higher you go up, there's not going to be that many African-Americans in your math because... they didn't really give a reason, but they just said how it's going to be dwindling, and so you can't get phased by the lack of African-Americans there, and you can't get intimidated or whatever.

TE: Okay. What do you think about that?

Benjamin: I guess I've taken that advice and I've used it. So – I don't get that intimidated, and I don't see that many African-Americans there because... I know all the people in the class have my same ability, so I shouldn't be intimidated . . . . Sometimes I feel like I have to try harder [in math], because not that many African-Americans are there with me, and so – it's good to have that title, like, that you are one of the few that were in that high math class, and stuff.

It is worth noting that Benjamin's parents were not alerting him to possible discrimination, or offering a reason for the lack of African-American students in higher-level math classes, but were trying to encourage their son to persist even when other African-American students did not. Benjamin likely saw the merit in his parents' message, especially when he saw with his own eyes the dwindling numbers of African-Americans in his math classes each year. Thus, for Benjamin, this racial-mathematical socialization message served as a support to help him cope with

[3] The 40-item TERS measure assesses racial socialization messages that African-American adolescents have heard from their parents; because racial socialization was not used in the analyses, this measure is not described in detail in this chapter.
[4] The original sample included non-African-American students as well; while they completed the YSRM also, they were assigned to complete the RMAS as their second questionnaire because the other two questionnaires were oriented towards African-American youth. Only African-American youth were included in the analysis presented here.

the challenge of being one of few African-American students in his high-level math class. Upon hearing this message, Benjamin engaged in adaptive coping: he took his parents' advice to not be intimidated, and consequently perceived himself as equally capable compared to the other students. This coping process helped to sustain his positive mathematical identity.

Racism and Discrimination in a Math Setting – Structural
Merlin, a 9th grade student at Obsidian school, described hearing a story about his grandmother's experience in a segregated math classroom. Merlin did well in math and perceived himself as good at math, especially as compared to other students in his class.

TE: Okay. Alright. Has your mom or anyone else – teachers, neighbors, anybody – ever told you a story about math that had anything to do with race?

Merlin: My grandmother, actually. She said. . .she had been in a kind of. . . what do you call those?. . . The two-race schools, but back then it was all racism, no blacks. . .

TE: Oh, like a segregated school.

Merlin: There we go, yeah. And they had, like, Whites in the left half and the Blacks in the right half. And in the right half, she *clearly* stated this – it was *always dirty*. And no matter how hard you tried, it would always stay dirty. And I don't remember if she said this, but she might have said, I'm not sure – that the janitors never came over on that side. Because the way I'm picturing, the way she said it, was all clean, not sparkly clean on the left side, but still kinda clean, you could walk, you could see the floor. Here was all dingy and, graffiti everywhere, and – I didn't like it, but. She also said that the textbooks for math were easy. . . extremely easy – they were the same for a few years, and then they finally went up a little, and continued like that. I didn't like that . . . . It kinda made me feel sad, because that means that a lot of people didn't really get a whole lot of education in math, and. . .not even sure about the other subjects, but. . .

TE: Do you ever think about that story?

Merlin: Yes, a lot.

TE: What do you think about, when you think about it?

Merlin: I mean, some people would complain – this is from her story – some people would complain and try to get other books, and they'd be kicked out because they wouldn't listen, or something . . . . And every time I think about it, I just think, 'Why?' 'Why??' Every time, I just keep repeating, 'Why?' I don't even know, it's just . . . unbelievable.

His grandmother's story seemed to affect Merlin greatly, and he continually wondered why this kind of segregation and discrimination occurred. He felt sad that so many people did not receive much education in math as a result of systemic racial discrimination, and that if they

complained about their situation, they would be expelled from school for insubordination. Merlin did not seem to have a way to reconcile for himself why the nation would subject these Black students to such conditions. As a result, this racial-mathematical socialization served as a net stress level challenge for Merlin. He engaged in some maladaptive coping, keeping the story to himself and not even discussing it with his younger sister, but he also felt thankful for his own educational opportunities as a result of hearing this story. The effect on his emergent identity is a bit unclear at this point in his life, but this racial-mathematical socialization story did contribute to his understanding of racism and racial discrimination.

Racism and Racial Discrimination in A Math Setting – Individual
Rashida, a 10th grade student at Obsidian school, recalled hearing a story about her mother being called a racial slur by a student during a math class.

Rashida: [My mom] said when she was younger. . . one time she didn't get this problem, and [a White girl named] Leah started cursing at her and calling her all types of n-words and all this stuff cause she didn't get it. She said 'Oh, you a stupid n, you this, you that.

TE: How do you feel about that?

Rashida: I don't know. If it'd been me, it wouldn't have been me. I wouldn't let her pass. This was like 1st grade, but I wouldn't let her pass . . . . I wouldn't let her go. [If] somebody call me a n-word, if they White, they gettin' an ordinary beat-down . . . . Yeah, something different. I'm gonna kick them in they face . . . . I'm not *gonna*. But . . . they'll get tore up – they gonna be red for days . . . . You don't call me a n-word and get away with it. [My mom] says if she was her, back then as she is now, she'd have beat the little girl up. But she says that you can't – you gotta learn this from the past.

TE: What did she do at the time?

Rashida: Nothing – she just sat back, didn't do nothing. She said she didn't do nothing about it but tell the teacher about it and the teacher didn't say nothing about it.

In sharing this story with her, Rashida's mother seemed to be trying to inform her about mistreatment of Blacks in the past, including the use of derogatory names. Although it took place during a math class (taught by a Black teacher who ignored the insults), this particular story did not seem inherently connected to mathematics; it could have easily happened during the teaching of any subject matter. Consequently, this racial-mathematical socialization story likely did not serve as either a challenge or a support in terms of Rashida's racialized beliefs about mathematics or in terms of her self-confidence in mathematics. Rashida responded angrily to her mother's story; this was an adaptive coping response in that she did not internalize the derogatory name but instead imagined defending herself against such an offense. Her coping response likely contributed to, or even reflected, her emergent racial identity.

Asians' High Performance in Math

Wendy, a 10th grade student at Galena school, briefly described a message that she had heard from her school friends about Asian students being universally good at math:

TE: All right. Did your parents or any other people tell you any stories about math that had to do with race or experiences with math that had. . .?

Wendy: Not usually. But. . . like with friends you be like, 'Oh, the Asian students know how to do math.' You go over to them and ask them how to do certain problems or something like that.

TE: Do they usually know how to do them?

Wendy: Yeah, most of them. . . depending on who the person is. But usually they do.

Unlike other types of racial-mathematical socialization messages and stories, the message Wendy reported was brought up by her peers rather than parents or older family members. This message seemed to serve as both a net stress-level challenge and support, in that it identified a source of mathematical assistance but called into question the mathematical capabilities of African-American students. Wendy seemed to take up this message and participate in its proliferation, a coping response that could be considered both adaptive and maladaptive (considering the dual nature of the message). Because Wendy seemed to agree with this message while recognizing that she knew students of other races (including African-Americans) who were good at math, it is unclear whether or how this message affected her emergent racial-mathematical identity.

Racial-mathematical socialization stories and messages seemed to primarily function as net stress level supports (or challenges) for youth. These supports and challenges were typically associated with reactive coping responses, which in turn contributed to the youths' emergent racial, mathematical, and/or racial-mathematical identities. A large proportion of the racial-mathematical socialization stories and messages reported seemed to inform the youth about racism or racial discrimination, such as with Merlin and Rashida. In each of these cases, the youth were angry, sad, and/or surprised that their relative had experienced such discrimination. Three youths were told about the strategies that were used to cope with the discrimination, as well as the outcomes of those strategies. The youth who heard stories of this type did not seem to know what to think of them and did not typically report taking action or planning to take action as a result; they primarily reported negative emotional reactions that likely influenced their emergent racial and mathematical identities.

On the other hand, the message types reported by Benjamin and Wendy informed them about racial differences in math. Wendy's message informed her about a racial difference in math but did not explain the reason for the perception that Asian students are good in math. Benjamin's message was similar in that it addressed the dearth of African-Americans in upper-level math classes. However, instead of informing him about any type of discrimination that might have resulted in that racial imbalance, his parents gave him advice to cope with being one of very few African-Americans in math classes. Wendy and Benjamin did not report experiencing emotional reactions to the messages about racial differences, but instead reported adaptive coping responses that involved action. Benjamin reported feeling that he should try harder in math because few Black students can reach the level in math that he has, and Wendy was likely to approach Asian students for assistance with math as a result of her message. Thus, it seems that youths' coping responses may differ for messages or stories about math that describe discrimination or racism than for messages that describe racial differences in math. Messages and stories about racial differences in mathematics may tend to result in changes in youths' actions, while messages and stories about math-related discrimination may tend to result primarily in negative emotional responses, at least while the youth have not experienced similar discrimination. It is possible that upon experiencing math-related discrimination, racial-mathematical socialization messages about discrimination may serve primarily as supports to help youth cope with this type of discrimination; however, because very few of the youth in this study reported having already experienced racial-mathematical discrimination, the support provided by these messages may only become evident as these youth progress further through school.

Racial-Mathematical Beliefs

To understand more about the socialization around math and race that youth receive, in this section we analyze the responses to the stereotype categories on the survey. Responses to these questions provide information about youths' beliefs about these stereotypes or common beliefs regarding math and race, and may provide a glimpse into youths' socialization in this area, even though they do not directly indicate the messages that youth have received about these stereotypes and racialized math beliefs. These racial-mathematical beliefs likely serve as coping responses resulting from youths' net stress level challenges and supports (racial-mathematical socialization and personal experiences with math and race). They can also serve as net stress level challenges and supports themselves. For example, if an African-American boy believes that African-Americans cannot do advanced mathematics, this belief may counteract a support such as a math teacher who tries

Table 1. Cross-tabulation of stereotype items on Black math performance

			Statement: 'Adults of my race use math in their daily lives'			Total
			disagree or strongly disagree	not sure	agree or strongly agree	
Statement: 'People of my race are typically good at math'	disagree or strongly disagree	count	5	8	23	36
		expected count	1.8	7.5	26.7	36.0
		total	3.1%	4.9%	14.1%	22.1%
		Std. residual	2.4	0.2	−0.7	
	not sure	count	1	21	67	89
		expected count	4.4	18.6	66.1	89.0
		total	6%	12.9%	41.1%	54.6%
		Std. residual	−1.6	0.6	0.1	
	agree or strongly agree	count	2	5	31	38
		expected count	1.9	7.9	28.2	38.0
		total	1.2%	3.1%	19.0%	23.3%
		Std. residual	0.1	−1.0	0.5	
	total	count	8	34	121	163
		expected count	8.0	34.0	121.0	163.0
		total	4.9%	20.9%	74.2%	100.0%

to get him to work harder because she knows he can do well in math.

Black Math Performance
Almost 80% of African-American youth agreed with at least one of the statements regarding African-Americans' experiences with math, while only 23.8% disagreed with one or both statements ('Adults of my race use math in their daily lives' and 'People of my race are typically good at math'). This suggests that the majority of African-American youth have positive views about African-Americans' experiences with math, particularly regarding the use of math in real life. Table 1 shows that an overwhelming majority of African-American youth, almost 75%, thought that adults of their own race use math in their daily lives.

However, African-American youth were divided as to whether they perceived that people of their race were typically good at math, while more than half of youth were unsure how people of their race typically performed in math. This indicates that most African-American youth may not have been socialized to have particular beliefs about African-American math abilities, or that they had not yet come to their own conclusions about these abilities.

Racial Discrimination in Math
It seems that the African-American youth in our sample largely did not agree that African-Americans were necessarily held back in math because of race, and about half of the youth agreed that African-Americans were given as many opportunities to succeed in math as people of other races. Twenty to 32% of youth in the sample were unsure as to whether African-Americans face either blatant (i.e., were held back in math due to race) or subtle racial discrimination in math (i.e., not given as many opportunities as others to succeed, which could also be interpreted as not being given as much support or assistance as others). However, while less than 5% thought that African-Americans face this blatant racial discrimination in math, almost 30% thought that African-Americans face the more subtle racial discrimination in the field of mathematics. A cross-tabulation of the two questions on beliefs about discrimination against

Table 2. Cross-tabulation of stereotype items on racial discrimination in math

			Statement: 'Blacks/African-Americans are held back in math because of their race'			Total
			agree or strongly agree	not sure	disagree or strongly disagree	
Statement: 'Black people are given as many opportunities to succeed in mathematics as people of other races'	disagree or strongly disagree	count	4	17	28	49
		expected count	2.4	15.8	30.8	49.0
		total	2.4%	10.4%	17.1%	29.9%
		Std. residual	1.0	0.3	−0.5	
	not sure	count	1	16	15	32
		expected count	1.6	10.3	20.1	32.0
		total	6%	9.8%	9.1%	19.5%
		Std. residual	−0.4	1.8	−1.1	
	agree or strongly agree	count	3	20	60	83
		expected count	4.0	26.8	52.1	83.0
		total	1.8%	12.2%	36.6%	50.6%
		Std. residual	−0.5	−1.3	1.1	
	total	count	8	53	103	164
		expected count	8.0	53.0	103.0	164.0
		total	4.9%	32.3%	62.8%	100.0%

African-Americans in math (see table 2) showed that while 36.6% of African-American youth thought that African-Americans are not held back in math because of their race or given fewer opportunities to succeed in math as people of other races, only 2.4% of African-American youth perceived that African-Americans face both the subtle and overt types of discrimination in mathematics. This suggests a complicated picture of African-American youths' perception of racial discrimination in mathematics.

Thus, it seems that while many African-American youth believed that African-Americans have the same opportunities to succeed in math as other races and do not face any type of racism or discrimination in math, almost a third of African-American youth believed that while African-Americans do not face both unequal opportunity and being held back in math, they do face at least one of these types of discrimination in math. It is possible that many African-American 9th and 10th graders have not yet encountered life experiences that would lead them to believe that racial discrimination occurs in the field of mathematics. It is also possible that some youth have already experienced racial-mathematical discrimination, but have not yet perceived these experiences as discriminatory, and they may perceive their experiences differently in retrospect as adults. Some studies have shown that African-American adults do believe that racial discrimination was rampant in their own mathematical experiences throughout their elementary, secondary, and post-secondary education [McGee, 2009; Martin, 2000; 2006]. Additionally, African-American teenagers and adults (along with other racial minorities) have been found to experience daily racial microaggressions, situations in which they are unsure whether they are being discriminated against or treated unfairly because of their race; these microaggressions typically have negative psychological effects on the individual [e.g., see Sue, Capodilupo & Holder, 2008; Torres, Driscoll & Burrow, 2010]. It is possible that the frequency of racial micro-aggressions in their daily lives contributes to African-Americans' perceptions of racial discrimination in mathematics.

Table 3. Cross-tabulation of stereotype items on Black math student performance

			Statement: 'The popular Black students in my school don't do well in math'			Total
			agree or strongly agree	not sure	disagree or strongly disagree	
Statement: 'In my math classes, students of other races have gotten higher grades than Black students'	agree or strongly agree	count	15	31	11	57
		expected count	10.4	31.4	15.2	57.0
		total	9.1%	18.8%	6.7%	34.5%
		Std. residual	1.4	−0.1	−1.1	
	not sure	count	7	33	13	53
		expected count	9.6	29.2	14.1	53.0
		total	4.2%	20.0%	7.9%	32.1%
		Std. residual	−0.8	0.7	−0.3	
	disagree or strongly disagree	count	8	27	20	55
		expected count	10.0	30.3	14.7	55.0
		total	4.8%	16.4%	12.1%	33.3%
		Std. residual	−0.6	−0.6	1.4	
	total	count	30	91	44	165
		expected count	30.0	91.0	44.0	165.0
		total	18.2%	55.2%	26.7%	100.0%

Black Math Student Performance

Table 3 shows that while 9.1% of the African-American youth in our sample had distinctly negative views about Black math student performance, and 12.1% had distinctly positive views, the majority of youth were unsure to some degree about how the Black students in their school perform in math. Twenty-three percent had somewhat negative views, and 24.3% had somewhat positive views, with 11.5% having ambivalent (both positive and negative) views.

These findings suggest that among African-American youth, there is no single 'stereotypical' view of Black students' math performance, such as a belief among youth that popular African-American students do not do well in math classes, or that African-American students perform worse than students of other races in math. In fact, less than one-third of youth agreed with either statement. However, slightly less than one-third of youth thought that students of other races have earned higher math grades than African-American students in their math classes, which indicates that a sizeable proportion of youth may have seen evidence in their math classes that African-American students do not fare as well as students of other races in math.

Asian Performance in Math

African-American youth were widely distributed on the question about whether they believed that Asian Americans are better in math than people of other races. While 35.1% agreed or strongly agreed with this stereotype, 38.1% disagreed or strongly disagreed, and 25.0% were not sure how they felt. This is a very common stereotype, as the results suggest; however, a slight majority of youth disagreed with this stereotype, which suggests that many youth have known Asian American students who did not do well in math, or that they simply know some students of other races who they consider to be brilliant in math. Regardless of the reason, a large proportion of the youth did not seem to think that Asian-Americans have a monopoly on high math performance.

In the next section, we discuss the relationships between these racial-mathematical belief types and constructs of math attitudes and racial identity.

Relationships: Racial-Mathematical Beliefs and Identity
An analysis of bivariate correlations revealed no relationship between the racial-mathematical beliefs and math grades or between racial-mathematical beliefs and gender. However, we found relationships between racial-mathematical beliefs and math attitudes, as well as between racial-mathematical beliefs and racial identity constructs. In order to determine whether there were any differences by grade level, correlations were performed for the sample overall and then for 9th graders and 10th graders separately.

Racial-Mathematical Beliefs and Math Attitudes
Overall, we found that Black math student performance beliefs were positively correlated with perceived usefulness of math, indicating that youth who perceived math as useful were more likely to have positive beliefs about the math performance of African-American youth in their schools. This finding was maintained in the grade-level analysis, as it was found to be the case for both 9th and 10th grade African-American youth. Additionally, the overall analysis revealed that youth with higher effectance motivation in math tended to believe that African-Americans do not experience racial discrimination in math. The grade-level analysis showed that this relationship was only significant among 9th grade youth and the overall sample; this correlation was not significant for 10th graders. For 9th graders, youth with higher overall attitudes about math also tended to believe that African-Americans do not experience racial discrimination in math. This was not the case for 10th graders, for whom there was no significant association between math attitudes and beliefs about racial discrimination in math. Additionally, tenth grade African-American students with more positive overall attitudes about math, as well as higher confidence and effectance motivation, tended to disbelieve the stereotype that Asian-Americans were better in math than people of other races. For 9th graders, there was no such relationship. Together, these findings suggest that for African-American youth, having positive attitudes towards math is associated with holding positive beliefs about Black math student performance at one's school, rejecting the stereotype of Asian Americans as better in math than others, and perceiving a lack of racial-mathematical discrimination against African-Americans.

Racial-Mathematical Beliefs and Racial Identity
We found that endorsement of the stereotype that Asian Americans are better in math than people of other races was associated with higher Public Regard and Assimilationism scores. This means that African-American youth with positive perceptions of other people's views of African-Americans tend to believe that Asian Americans are better in math than people of other races. Additionally, African-

American youth who believe that African-Americans should assimilate into the majority White culture tend to believe this stereotype. From the grade level analysis, the correlation with Assimilationist beliefs was found to be significant only for 9th graders, and the correlation with Public Regard was significant only in the overall analysis. It is possible that African-American youth who think that others have positive views of their racial group, as well as those who believe that African-Americans should assimilate into White culture, tend to perceive education and academics as completely meritocratic (and thus free of external societal forces), and as a result may be more likely to tacitly accept societal views about Asian-Americans and math.

Overall, and for both 9th and 10th graders separately, having high Public Regard was associated with positive beliefs about African-American adults' use of and performance in math. High Public Regard was also found to be associated with lower perceptions of racial discrimination in math in the overall sample; this relationship was significant only for 10th graders in the grade-level analysis. Having high Public and Private Regard was associated with positive Black racial math performance beliefs in the overall sample, meaning that African-American youth with positive views of African-Americans as well as positive perceptions of others' views of African-Americans tended to believe that African-Americans were typically good at math and used math regularly. In the grade-level analysis, the relationship between Private Regard and Black racial math performance beliefs was evident for 10th graders only.

It is noteworthy that youth with positive views of African-Americans, as well as those who perceive that others have positive views of African-Americans, tended to believe that African-Americans were typically good at math and used math regularly. This suggests that general self-perceptions and beliefs about others' perceptions of one's own racial group carry over into mathematics. If an African-American girl perceives African-Americans generally in a negative light, she is likely to also perceive African-Americans' math use and performance negatively, which may result in her putting forth less effort in math class, reducing her mathematical aspirations, and developing a negative mathematical identity.

In the overall sample, espousing Humanism beliefs was associated with lower Black math student performance beliefs, meaning that African-American youth who believe that one should focus on individual characteristics rather than on group characteristics such as race tended to perceive that African-American students in their school performed worse in math than students of other races. The grade-level analysis showed this relationship as significant only for 10th graders. Additionally, among 10th graders, espousing Humanism beliefs was associated with holding negative beliefs about African-Americans adults' use of and performance in math.

Discussion

Overt racial-mathematical socialization messages and stories, while not heard by all African-American youths, are rather common. This type of socialization can serve as a support for African-American youth, in that it can prepare them to cope with net stress-level challenges such as racial discrimination in math settings or being the only African-American in a high-level math class. However, racial-mathematical socialization messages and stories can also serve as a challenge for youth, especially if the messages cause the youth to question their own mathematical abilities or chances of success.

Only youths with positive or somewhat positive attitudes about math reported hearing racial-mathematical messages and stories. The parents and significant others of these youth may purposely expose them to this type of socialization because they are likely to take advanced math classes (and thus are more likely than other youth to encounter the challenges of being the only African-American or experiencing overt racial discrimination in an advanced math class). It is unfortunate that youth with negative mathematical identities did not receive this type of socialization, as racial-mathematical socialization messages that focus on African-Americans persisting in math would likely serve as a support that could help to counteract the challenge of their negative mathematical experiences. Alternatively, messages about discrimination or racism in math settings might result in maladaptive coping responses among youth with negative feelings about math.

There seems to be no overarching negative stereotypical view of Black students' math performance, as African-American youth were evenly split in their views about the math performance of African-American students relative to youth of other races at their schools. Additionally, African-American youth were quite varied in their beliefs about the math performance of Asian Americans compared to people of other races. This suggests that many African-American youth are not blindly accepting societal stereotypes about race and math, regardless of whether they describe Asian Americans or African-Americans. Some African-Americans may even use coping responses that enhance their mathematical achievement when faced with negative stereotypes [McGee, 2009]. On the other hand, a sizeable percentage of African-American youth do seem to accept these stereotypes. In coping with these stereotypes, youth likely rely on the socialization they receive from their parents and friends, which can impact their perceptions of their own capabilities in mathematics, and thereby affect their emergent mathematical and racial-mathematical identities.

The findings regarding beliefs about racial-mathematical discrimination may reflect familial or societal-level socialization regarding racial discrimination in math settings and/or the dearth of African-Americans in positions that require high levels of mathematical preparation. Many of the interviewed youth did not recall hearing any racial-mathematical socialization messages or stories, but of those who did, the majority of these messages and stories discussed discrimination or racism in math settings. This suggests that such socialization serves as a net stress-level support or challenge that impacts youths' beliefs about race and mathematics.

Ninth graders' overall math attitudes and effectance motivation were related to their attitudes about racial discrimination in math. 10th graders' overall math attitudes, effectance motivation, and confidence in math were related to their attitudes about Asians' performance in math. Perhaps by 10th grade, youths' math attitudes no longer affect their perceptions of whether African-Americans face discrimination in math; perceptions of racial-mathematical discrimination in older youth may be affected more by their (more developed) beliefs about race and racial discrimination more broadly rather than their personal feelings about math. These findings also suggest that around 10th grade, a connection exists between math attitudes and perceptions about Asian-Americans' performance in math. This may be a result of increased difficulty in the mathematical concepts that youth encounter as they get older; 10th graders may begin to perceive evidence of Asian-American students outperforming students of other races (or not) in their own math classes as these classes become more difficult and more students begin to struggle with the math content. However, the timing of this connection may depend on the timing of youths' first extensive interactions with Asian-American students; African-American youth who attend racially integrated elementary or middle schools may perceive Asian-American students' math performance as advanced (or equal to others') at a much earlier point in time than might African-American youth who first encounter Asian-American students during high school or college. Alternatively, 10th grade African-American youth who experience significant difficulty with the math content as they get older may turn to existing societal stereotypes about Asian Americans' high math performance as a maladaptive coping strategy to reconcile their own struggles with math. However, it is unlikely that youth only begin to develop racialized beliefs about mathematics in high school; future research should target elementary and middle school children as well to investigate relationships between beliefs about math and race over time.

Racial identity constructs were more closely related to racial-mathematical beliefs for 10th graders than for 9th graders. As racial identity tends to be more developed in older adolescents, this finding is expected, and it suggests that during adolescence, one's developing racial identity becomes increasingly related to one's racialized beliefs about math. Future research should examine this relationship more closely.

Public Regard was particularly closely related to racial-mathematical beliefs, as it was associated with three of the four racial-mathematical belief types for the overall sample; it was not related to perceptions of Black student math performance. This relationship may be due to the similarity between the constructs of Public Regard and the different racial-mathematical belief types, as most of the racial-mathematical belief types studied here rely on youths' views of other people's perceptions of African-Americans. In this vein, it is surprising that Private Regard was not more closely related to most of the racial-mathematical belief types in the overall sample. It may be the case that discussions about Blacks in the larger society, at home, or in school, though strongly influencing youth, are coded in such a way that youth may only cognitively connect some of them to mathematics.

As with all research that relies on surveys for assessing youths' beliefs, there are limitations in how thoroughly we are able to uncover and understand these youths' racial-mathematical beliefs. Because surveys ask for agreement or disagreement with statements that are phrased in a particular manner, youths' responses may only provide abstract beliefs (beliefs that are based on abstract ideas about the way things should be) rather than concrete beliefs, which are based on the lived experiences of those around the youth [Mickelson, 1990]. Although the interviews served to provide a deeper understanding of some youths' socialization messages, beliefs, and coping processes used in negotiating the risks and protective factors, challenges and supports they faced, due to the relatively short duration of the interviews, we could only scratch the surface in uncovering these understandings. For this reason, it is important that future research uses both qualitative and quantitative approaches to investigate African-American youths' racial-mathematical beliefs, experiences, socialization, coping responses, and identities.

English-Clarke · Slaughter-Defoe · Martin

Conclusion

Racial-mathematical socialization may serve as a special support for youth rather than just an additional context for racial socialization. Youth who hear these racial-mathematical socialization stories or messages may develop a deeper and more complex understanding of the far-reaching effects of discrimination, the youth-relevant contexts in which discrimination can occur, and the racial imbalances that they may perceive as they reach higher levels of mathematics. These socialization messages may help to shape the coping responses that youth employ to cope with the challenges posed by the various mathematical and racial-mathematical experiences that they encounter over time.

While negative racial-mathematical stereotypes seem to be endorsed by many African-American youth, a sizeable proportion of youth reject the stereotypes that reflect negatively on African-Americans' mathematical abilities. As youths' racial identities develop, their understandings about race seem to increasingly affect their racial-mathematical beliefs. This suggests that in order to positively influence African-American youths' racial-mathematical beliefs, parents, teachers, and society at large must socialize youth in such a way that encourages them to believe in their own mathematical potential as African-Americans. We must also provide socialization messages and stories that help youth to recognize and overcome racial discrimination in math or other racial barriers to mathematical success that they may encounter.

References

Bennett, M.D. (2006). Culture and context: A study of neighborhood effects on racial socialization and ethnic identity content in a sample of African-American adolescents. *Journal of Black Psychology, 32,* 479–500.

Brown, T.L., Linver, M.R., Evans, M., & DeGennaro, D. (2009). African-American parents' racial and ethnic socialization and adolescent academic grades: Teasing out the role of gender. *Journal of Youth Adolescence, 38,* 214–227.

Brown, T.L., Linver, M.R., & Evans, M. (2010). The role of gender in the racial and ethnic socialization of African-American adolescents. *Youth & Society, 41,* 357–381.

Bynum, M.S., Burton, E.T., & Best, C. (2007). Racism experiences and psychological functioning in African-American college freshmen: Is racial socialization a buffer? *Cultural Diversity and Ethnic Minority Psychology, 13,* 64–71.

Chatman, C.M., Eccles, J.S., & Malanchuk, O. (2005). Identity negotiation in everyday settings. In J. Downey, J.S. Eccles, & C.M. Chatman (Eds.), *Navigating the future: Social identity, coping, and life tasks* (pp. 116–139).

Cross, W.E. (1991). *Shades of black: Diversity in African-American identity.* Chapter 6: Rethinking Nigrescence (pp. 189–223). Philadelphia: Temple University Press.

Dweck, C. (1999). Self-theories: Their role in motivation, personality, and development. Philadelphia: Psychology Press.

Eccles, J. (1997). User-friendly science and mathematics: Can it interest girls and minorities in breaking through the middle school wall? In D. Johnson (Ed.), *Minorities and girls in school: Effects on achievement and performance. Leaders in psychology. Vol. 1* (pp. 65–104). Thousand Oaks: Sage Publications, Inc.

English-Clarke, T.L. (2011). Things my family told me about math: African-American youths' perception and use of racial and mathematical socialization messages. Doctoral Dissertation, University of Pennsylvania.

Fennema, E., & Sherman, J.A. (1976). Mathematics attitudes scales: Instruments designed to measure attitudes toward the learning of mathematics by females and males. *Journal for Research in Mathematics Education, 7,* 324–326.

Gordon, B. (1990). The necessity of African-American epistemology for educational theory and practice. *Journal of Education, 172,* 88–106.

Helms, J. (2007). Some better practices for measuring racial and ethnic identity constructs. *Journal of Counseling Psychology.* Special Issue: Racial and ethnic identity theory, measurement, and research in counseling psychology: Present status and future directions, *54,* 235–246.

Hughes, D., & Chen, L. (1997). When and what parents tell children about race: An examination of race-related socialization among African-American families. *Applied Developmental Science, 1,* 200–214.

Hughes, D., et al. (2006). Parents' ethnic-racial socialization practices: A review of research and directions for future study. *Developmental Psychology, 42,* 747–770.

Jackson, K.J. (2009). The social construction of youth and mathematics: The case of a fifth grade classroom. In D.B. Martin (Ed.), *Mathematics teaching, learning, and liberation in the lives of Black children* (pp. 175–199). New York, NY, US: Routledge/Taylor & Francis Group.

Lee, C.D., Spencer, M.B., & Harpalani, V. (2003). 'Every shut eye ain't sleep': Studying how people live culturally. *Educational Researcher, 32,* 6–13.

Martin, D. (1997). Mathematics socialization and identity among African-Americans: Community forces, school forces, and individual agency. Doctoral Dissertation, University of California, Berkeley.

Martin, D. (2000). Mathematics success and failure among African-American youth: The roles of sociohistorical context, community forces, school influence, and individual agency. Mahwah: Lawrence Erlbaum Associates.

Martin, D.B. (2006). Mathematics learning and participation as racialized forms of experience: African-American parents speak on the struggle for mathematics literacy. *Mathematical Thinking and Learning, 8,* 197–229.

Martin, D.B. (2007). Mathematics learning and participation in African-American context: The co-construction of identity in two intersecting realms of experience. In N. Nasir & P. Cobb (Eds.), *Improving access to mathematics: Diversity and equity in the classroom* (pp. 146–158). New York: Teachers College Press.

Martin, D.B. (2009). Liberating the production of knowledge about African-American children and mathematics. In D.B. Martin (Ed.), *Mathematics teaching, learning, and liberation in the lives of Black children* (pp. 3–36). New York: Routledge/Taylor & Francis Group.

McGee, E., & Martin, D. (2011). From the hood to being hooded: A case study of a Black male PhD. *Journal of African-American Males, 2,* 46–65.

McGee, E.O. (2010). Race, identity, and resilience: Black college students negotiating success in mathematics and engineering. Doctoral Dissertation, University of Illinois at Chicago.

Mickelson, R.A. (1990). The attitude-achievement paradox among Black adolescents. *Sociology of Education, 63,* 44–61.

Muuss, R.E. (1996). *Theories of adolescence* (6th ed.). New York, NY: McGraw Hill.

Nasir, N.S., & Saxe, G.B. (2003). Ethnic and academic identities: a cultural practice perspective on emerging tensions and their management in the lives of minority students. *Educational Researcher, 32,* 14–18.

Neblett, E.W., et al. (2008). Patterns of racial socialization and psychological adjustment: Can parental communications about race reduce the impact of racial discrimination? *Journal of Research on Adolescence, 18,* 477–515.

Nicholls, J.G. (1984). Achievement motivation: Conceptions of ability, subjective experience, task choice, and performance. *Psychological Review, 91,* 328–346.

Oyserman, D., Gant, L., & Ager, J. (1995). A socially contextualized model of African-American identity: Possible selves and school persistence. *Journal of Personality and Social Psychology, 69,* 1216–1232.

Phinney, J.S., & Alipuria, L.L. (1990). Ethnic identity in college students from four ethnic groups. *Journal of Adolescence, 13,* 171–183.

Phinney, J.S., & Chavira, V. (1995). Parental ethnic socialization and adolescent coping with problems related to ethnicity. *Journal of Research on Adolescence, 5,* 31–53.

Phinney, J.S., & Ong, A.D. (2007). Conceptualization and measurement of ethnic identity: Current status and future directions. *Journal of Counseling Psychology, 54,* 271–291.

Scottham, K.M., Sellers, R.M., & Nguyen, H.X. (2008). A measure of racial identity in African-American adolescents: The development of the Multidimensional Inventory of Black Identity – Teen. *Cultural Diversity and Ethnic Minority Psychology, 14,* 297–306.

Seaton, E.K., Scottham, K.M., & Sellers, R.M. (2006). The status model of racial identity development in African-American adolescents: Evidence of structure, trajectories, and well-being. *Child Development, 77,* 1416–1426.

Sellers, R.M., Rowley, S.A.J., Chavous, T.M., Shelton, J.N., & Smith, M.A. (1997). Multidimensional inventory of Black identity: A preliminary investigation of reliability and construct validity. *Journal of Personality and Social Psychology, 73,* 805–815.

Sellers, R.M., Smith, M.A., Shelton, J.N., Rowley, S.A.J., & Chavous, T.M. (1998). Multidimensional model of racial identity: A reconceptualization of African-American racial identity. *Personality and Social Psychology Review, 2,* 18–39.

Slaughter-Defoe, D. (1995). Revisiting the concept of socialization: Caregiving and teaching in the 90s – A personal perspective. *American Psychologist, 50,* 276–286.

Slaughter-Defoe, D., Johnson, D., & Spencer, M.B. (2009). Race and child development. In R. Shweder (Ed.), *The child: An encyclopedic companion* (pp. 801–806). Chicago: University of Chicago Press.

Spencer, M.B. (1995). Old issues and new theorizing about African-American youth: A phenomenological variant of ecological systems theory. In R.L. Taylor (Ed.), *Black youth: Perspectives on their status in the United States* (pp. 37–70). Westport: Praeger.

Spencer, J.A. (2009). Identity at the crossroads: Understanding the processes and forces that shape African-American success and struggle in mathematics. In D.B. Martin (Ed.), *Mathematics teaching, learning, and liberation in the lives of Black children* (pp. 200–230). New York: Routledge.

Spencer, M.B., & Markstrom-Adams, C. (1990). Identity processes among racial and ethnic minority children in America. *Child Development, 61,* 290–310.

Spencer, M.B., et al. (2006). Understanding vulnerability and resilience from a normative developmental perspective: Implications for racially and ethnically diverse youth. In D. Cicchetti & D.J. Cohen (Eds.), *Developmental psychopathology. Vol. 1: Theory and method* (pp. 627–672). Hoboken: Wiley.

Stevenson, H.C., Jr., Cameron, R., Herrero-Taylor, T., & Davis, G. (2002). Development of the teenager experience of racial socialization scale: Correlates of race-related socialization frequency from the perspective of black youth. *Journal of Black Psychology, 25,* 84–106.

Stevenson, H.C., Jr., & Davis, G.Y. (2004). Racial socialization. In R. Jones (Ed.), *Black psychology* (4th ed., pp. 353–381). Hampton, VA: Cobb and Henry.

Stinson, D.W. (2006). African-American male adolescents, schooling (and mathematics): Deficiency, rejection, and achievement. *Review of Educational Research, 76,* 477–506.

Stinson, D.W. (2009). Negotiating sociocultural discourses: The counter-storytelling of academically and mathematically successful African-American male students. In D.B. Martin (Ed.), *Mathematics teaching, learning, and liberation in the lives of Black children* (pp. 265–288). New York: Routledge/Taylor & Francis Group.

Stinson, D.W. (2011). When the 'burden of acting White' is not a burden: School success and African-American male students. *Urban Review, 43,* 43–65.

Sue, D.W., Capodilupo, C.M., & Holder, A.M.B. (2008). Racial microaggressions in the life of African-Americans. *Professional Psychology: Research and Practice, 39,* 329–336.

Tatum, B.D. (1997). 'Why are all the Black kids sitting together in the cafeteria?' New York: Basic Books.

Tillman, L.C. (2002). Culturally sensitive research approaches: An African-American perspective. *Educational Researcher, 31,* 3–12.

Torres, L., Driscoll, M.W., & Burrow, A.L. (2010). Racial microaggressions and psychological functioning among highly-achieving African-Americans: A mixed-methods approach. *Journal of Social and Clinical Psychology, 29,* 1074–1099.

Wigfield, A., & Eccles, J. (2000). Expectancy-value theory of achievement motivation. *Contemporary Educational Psychology. Special Motivation and the Educational Process, 25,* 68–81.

Yip, T., Seaton, E.K., & Sellers, M. (2006). African-American racial identity across the lifespan: Identity status, identity content, and depressive symptoms. *Child Development, 77,* 1504–1517.

Dr. Traci L. English-Clarke (PhD 2011, University of Pennsylvania) earned her doctorate in Teaching, Learning, and Curriculum, with distinction for her dissertation on the racial and mathematical socialization messages received by African-American youth. A former Spencer Foundation fellow, she graduated cum laude from Harvard University with a BA in Sociology. Her research interests are mathematics education, mathematical identity, mathematical socialization, racial identity, racial socialization, and family influences on youth identity and learning. She is interested in developing interventions that enable youth of all races to develop a sustained appreciation for mathematics throughout adolescence.

Dr. Danny Bernard Martin (PhD 1997, University of California, Berkeley, Calif., USA) is Professor of Education and Mathematics at the University of Illinois at Chicago. Prior to coming to UIC, he was Instructor and Professor in the Department of Mathematics at Contra Costa College for 14 years, serving as Chair for 3 years, and was a National Academy of Education/Spencer Foundation Postdoctoral Fellow from 1998–2000. Dr. Martin's research focuses on understanding the salience of race and identity in Black learners' mathematical experiences. He is the author of Mathematics Success and Failure among African-American Youth (2000, Lawrence Erlbaum Associates) and editor of Mathematics Teaching, Learning, and Liberationin the Lives of Black Children [2009, Routledge].

Dr. Diana T. Slaughter-Defoe (PhD 1968, University of Chicago) received her doctorate from the Committee on Human Development in developmental and clinical psychology, and is presently the Constance E. Clayton Professor Emerita in the Graduate School of Education at the University of Pennsylvania. Her research interests have included culture, primary education, and home-school relations facilitating in-school academic achievement. Since retirement, she has also edited: *Black Educational Choice: Assessing the Private and Public Alternatives to K-12 Public Schools* [Praeger, 2011] with colleagues, and *Messages for Educational Leadership: The Constance E. Clayton Lectures, 1998–2007* [Peter Lang Publishers, 2012]. She is presently writing a memoir about her career that spanned 40-plus years in academia and higher education.

T.L. English-Clarke
52391 Liberty Mills Ct.
Granger, IN 46530(USA)
Tel. +1 574 383–5557
E-Mail tenglish88@gmail.com

Commentary

Slaughter-Defoe DT (ed): Racial Stereotyping and Child Development.
Contrib Hum Dev. Basel, Karger, 2012, vol 25, pp 80–82

'What Do Race and Math Have to Do with Each Other?' Relationships between Racial-Mathematical Socialization, Mathematical Identity, and Racial Identity

Commentary on English-Clarke, Slaughter-Defoe, and Martin

Ebony McGee

National Science Foundation Minority Postdoctoral Fellow, Scientific Careers and Research Development Group, Northwestern University, Department of Faculty Affairs, Feinberg School of Medicine, Chicago, Ill., USA

Clearly, the authors have done their homework, incorporating traditional mathematics education paradigms with literature on socialization (parental, racial, and mathematics) and identity (developmental, racial, gender) to explore African-American early high schoolers' mathematics identities and their relationships to racialized experiences and beliefs. From a multidisciplinary perspective of *racial-mathematical socialization,* this mixed methods study combined survey data of 168 9th and 10th graders with in-depth information gathered from 35- to 45-min interviews of 28 of these students, taking a route that incorporates scholarship outside of the traditional mathematics education paradigm.

Issues of identity have been increasingly important in emergent mathematics education literature to understanding the mindset of mathematics students, particularly of marginalized students of color [e.g., Ellington, 2006; Martin, 2006a, b; Nasir, 2002; Spencer, 2009; Stinson, 2009]. Looking at identity through multiple lenses and investigating it via *Phenomenological Variant of Ecological Systems Theory* (PVEST), these authors have provided a robust justification for the exploration of narrative storytelling as a means to better understand the development of racial-mathematical identity. However, I would have hoped for more concrete linkages between PVEST and the results, for example, the illumination of risk and protective factors beyond adult-driven racial socialization practices, which may have contributed to the development of students' thoughts, beliefs, and subsequent actions.

Interestingly, English-Clarke and her colleague Martin have both uncovered an historical legacy of racialized experiences in mathematics, conveyed through storytelling, experiences that have helped to prepare these students to cope with discrimination in math settings. The students in this study also expressed positive beliefs about African American adults' engagement in mathematics and perceived the discipline as a useful one. Issues of developmental changes between the 9th and 10th graders, rarely noted in most traditional mathematics education studies, were given special attention. For example, awareness of racial stereotypes and other forms of racial discrimination might be more evident to 10th than to 9th graders. However, delving further into the school and community environments could have provided additional information on how early exposure to racialized experiences may also have played a role in how these students perceived and coped with racial mathematical awareness issues.

Because context matters, it would have been helpful to know more about the study's details, such as: (a) expanding the brief description of the metropolitan northeastern city where the study was conducted; (b) the career or college aspirations of the respondents, and (c) the racial make-up of their schools and neighborhoods. These factors could have offered greater insight into the research findings. Other recent research on this topic demonstrates that the racial make-up of schools and neighborhoods can play extremely important role in how students receive, and, in turn, process and develop racialized coping strategies. Indeed, coping strategies are, in part, a function of the larger environment and the prior exposure of students to racialized experiences [McGee, 2009; McGee & Beale Spencer, in press].

The authors convincingly provided a plethora of research to make a strong case for the use of mathematical-racial identity, mathematical racial socialization, and a few other developmentally and socially relevant perspectives. As I was very invested in this study, I was willing to wait to absorb the results. However, although a consolidated synthesis of this complex literature may be a difficult exercise, it may ultimately be necessary to provide a quicker path to the results.

The racial mathematical stories used in this study provide evidence of the long history of African Americans being blatantly denied equal opportunities in mathematics. However, due to the subtle nature of the current racialized practices, this study could have shown a more detailed scenario of how current-day racism can evolve into insidious covert practices and policies. Nevertheless, this study adds intellectual depth to current understandings of how African Americans students receive and process messages about their engagement in mathematics, processes that are dependent on their level of development, and how they see themselves, individually and within the larger society.

References

Ellington, R. (2006). Having their say: Eight high-achieving African-American undergraduate mathematics majors discuss their success and persistence in mathematics. Unpublished doctoral dissertation. University of Maryland, College Park.

Martin, D. (2006a). Mathematics learning and participation as racialized forms of experience: African American parents speak on the struggle for mathematics literacy. *Mathematical Thinking and Learning, 8,* 197–229.

Martin, D. (2006b). Mathematics learning and participation in African American context: The co-construction of identity in two intersecting realms of experience. In N. Nasir & P. Cobb (Eds.), *Diversity, equity, and access to mathematical ideas* (pp. 146–158). New York: Teachers College Press.

McGee, E.O. (2009). Race, identity, and resilience: Black college students negotiating success in mathematics and engineering. Unpublished doctoral dissertation, University of Illinois, Chicago.

McGee, E.O., & Spencer, M.B. (in press). Going from all Black to predominately White: The tumultuous transition of low SES Black students to PWIs. To appear. In C.C. Yeakey (Ed.), *Urban marginality: Youth, cities and neighborhoods in transition.*

Nasir, N.S. (2002). Identity, goals, and learning: Mathematics in cultural practice. In N. Nasir & P. Cobb (Eds.), *Mathematical thinking and learning, 4,* 213–248.

Spencer, J. (2009). Identity at the crossroads: Understanding the practices and forces that shape African American success and struggle in mathematics. In D. Martin (Ed.), *Mathematics teaching, learning, and liberation in the lives of Black children*. London: Routledge.

Stinson, D. (2009). Negotiating sociocultural discourses: The counter-storytelling of academically and mathematically successful African American male students. In D. Martin (Ed.), *Mathematics teaching, learning, and liberation in the lives of Black children*. London: Routledge.

Ebony McGee, Mathematics Education, PhD
Scientific Careers and Research Development Group, Northwestern University
Department of Faculty Affairs
Feinberg School of Medicine, Rubloff 12
420 E. Superior Ave.
Chicago, IL 60611–3152 (USA)
Tel. +1 312 503 2959
E-Mail ebony-mcgee@northwestern.edu

Dr. Ebony McGee (PhD 2009, University of Illinois at Chicago) is a National Science Foundation postdoctoral fellow at Northwestern University, with the Scientific Careers and Research Development Group. Her postdoctoral research study investigates successful African-American, Asian-American, and Latino physical science and mathematics advanced college students and the role of stereotypes and other influences in their postsecondary career and academic decision-making. More generally, her research focuses on the role of racial stereotypes in mathematics and science educational and career attainment, resiliency, and identity development and formation in mathematically high-achieving marginalized students of color.

Commentary

Slaughter-Defoe DT (ed): Racial Stereotyping and Child Development.
Contrib Hum Dev. Basel, Karger, 2012, vol 25, pp 83–86

The Need to Incorporate Observations of Implicit Socialization in the Contexts of Everyday Life

Commentary on English-Clarke, Slaughter-Defoe, and Martin

Peggy J. Miller[a] · Jeana R. Bracey[b]

[a]Department of Psychology, University of Illinois, Champaign-Urbana, Ill., and [b]Connecticut Center for Effective Practice of the Child Health and Development Institute of Connecticut, Farmington, Conn., USA

English-Clarke and colleagues have written an intriguing chapter on the intersection of race and mathematics in the socialization and identity development of African-American adolescents. We begin our commentary with some overarching comments and then turn to specific issues related to the qualitative study of socialization.

General Comments

The authors adopt a theoretically sophisticated framework that envisions both socialization and identity formation as deeply social processes embedded in and shaped by multiple ecologies, including institutional and cultural contexts and societal stereotypes of race, ethnicity, class, and gender. We applaud their goal of developing a more richly contextualized understanding of these fundamental processes. But given this grounding in contextual/ecological models, it is surprising that English-Clarke and colleagues provide so little description of the worlds that their participants inhabited. For example, did they attend public or private schools? What were the racial/ethnic demographics of their schools and neighborhoods? How did students and their parents perceive the racial climate of the school

and community? These kinds of details are particularly relevant because the authors define racial socialization in terms of efforts to prepare minority children to succeed in a hostile environment; this implies that parents might adapt their socializing messages and children might 'hear' those messages differently, depending on the racial/ethnic composition of the school and community and the history of race relations therein [e.g., Burton & Jarrett, 2000; Jarrett, 2003; Mattison & Aber, 2007; Pattillo-McCoy, 1999; Stevenson, McNeil, Herrero-Taylor & Davis, 2005].

Another strength of the study is the attention to individuals' *perception* of socializing messages, a focus that is well suited to the developmental moment in question, namely early adolescence. As the authors point out, racial/ethnic identity is especially salient for African American and other minority youth, and exploration of racial/ethnic identity begins early [Tatum, 1997]. García Coll and Marks [2009] have shown that middle-school children from minority (immigrant) backgrounds can already map a nuanced landscape of self-applicable racial/ethnic labels. Thus, there is ample reason to enlist 9th and 10th graders as savvy interpreters of their own and others' experiences of socialization and identity.

Perhaps the most unusual and provocative feature of the chapter is the focus on the intersection between race and mathematics. By taking on this problem, the authors stake out new territory; much more attention has been given to racial/ethnic socialization with respect to literacy or academic achievement in general [Bracey, 2010; Carter-Black, 2003, 2005; Franklin, Boyd-Franklin & Draper, 2002; Dyson, 2003; Hughes et al., 2006; Steele & Aronson, 1998]. By the same token, it would be useful to have a more fully developed theoretical and practical rationale: Why study the socialization of math and race rather than science and race, or foreign languages and race, or any other academic domain? The authors mention the dearth of African Americans in fields that require advanced mathematical knowledge but do not develop this important point. Another practical reason to pay more attention to math might be the more stringent curricular standards in mathematics instituted by the No Child Left Behind legislation. From a theoretical standpoint, might there be much to be gained by exploring a domain which is not so racially/ethnically salient or subject to racial/ethnic stereotyping?

Studying Socialization Qualitatively

As researchers whose work deals with socialization and narrative, using primarily qualitative and ethnographic methods [e.g., Bracey, 2010; Hudley, Haight & Miller, 2003; Miller, Cho & Bracey, 2005; Miller et al., 2012], we direct the remainder of our comments to the interview component of this mixed-method study. By using a mixed method approach, the authors join a growing list of researchers with a contextualized vision of development who see the value of balancing breadth and generalizability, on the one hand, with depth and nuance, on the other [e.g., Duncan, Houston & Weisner, 2007; García Coll & Marks, 2009; Weisner, 2005]. The authors surveyed 168 African American students and then conducted interviews with a subset of 28 participants. The latter were asked whether they had ever heard a message or story about math that had to do with race or about race that had to do with math; they were also asked about their reactions to the message or story.

About one-third of the students reported messages or stories about race and math together, and nearly half of these had to do with racial discrimination in math. The stories that the authors present are fascinating! More examples would have been even better. The interviewers apparently had excellent rapport with the interviewees, who felt free to share the strong emotions that the stories evoked. One notable feature of the two discrimination stories excerpted in the chapter is that both invoke incidents of overt racial discrimination with no possibility of redress, incidents that the adolescent interviewees (Merlin and Rashida) heard from a parent or grandparent. In their narrative representations of these appalling events, Merlin and Rashida imply a temporal distance from their own experience: Rashida says that she would not have 'let her [the racist White girl] pass' and Merlin, more subtly, represents himself as incredulous, 'Every time [I think of the story], I just keep repeating.' 'Why?' I don't even know, it's just. . . unbelievable.' Our reading of these narrative texts is that math per se was somewhat incidental in these young narrators' interpretations of what happened to their relatives; they depicted schools in which racial injustice was systemic, encompassing not only math but also dirty classrooms, third-rate materials, and teachers who were deaf to racial slurs.

These examples raise many tantalizing questions, suggesting that it would be worthwhile to analyze the whole corpus of stories at a micro-level. For instance, did the other discrimination stories also refer to events from previous generations? Were stories constructed to establish a point about discrimination in math or a point about the totalizing nature of racial discrimination? And how do such analyses relate to the findings from the questionnaire component? Given that substantial within-group variation emerged in both component studies, it would be useful to examine the narrative and questionnaire findings side by side. Perhaps some of the variation in beliefs about whether African Americans face discrimination in math (the majority indicated that African Americans do not face discrimination in math, almost one-third were unsure) relates to whether family members of older generations shared discrimination stories with them. In light of the authors' phenomenological perspective, a closely related issue has to do with how such stories – which were clearly profoundly important, even indelible to some of these young people – inform the way they interpret their *own* experience. When older generations provide a personalized historical perspective on race and math, do adolescents use these stories to create a benchmark from which to judge the current state of affairs (e.g., the situation is so much better for me and my generation, discrimination is much more subtle than it used to be)?

A host of interesting studies could be undertaken to build upon and extend this work. Given the critical importance of the historical context in shaping the experiences of and scholarship about African American children [Slaughter-Defoe, Johnson & Spencer, 2009], it would be fascinating to examine the perspectives of multiple generations on race and math, interviewing young people, their parents, and grandparents. This would illuminate more fully the historical situatedness of views of discrimination and socialization, as refracted through personal experience. It could also shed additional light on the other two content areas that emerged in the interviews. For example, Benjamin's description of his parents' advice – not to be intimidated as he moves into higher-level math classes where there are fewer African Americans – invites the question of whether they had had similar experiences in math classes. A great deal could be learned by studying multiple generations in African American lineages of mathematically talented individuals. How have successive generations socialized their children and supported the development of strong identities as mathematically gifted African Americans?

So far, the comments in this section pertain only to those interviewees who reported hearing messages or stories involving math and race. But two-thirds of the students did *not* report such messages or stories. Does this mean that they experienced no socialization at the intersection of race and math? Definitely not. In their influential work on racial socialization, Boykin and Toms [1985] emphasized that most socialization is tacit, learned through everyday routines, interactions with parents, and consistent styles of behavior. Bracey's [2010] longitudinal ethnographic study of early racial socialization in two African American families supports this claim while also showing that parents were strongly and explicitly committed to promoting academic achievement, often using it as a vehicle for indexing race more subtly. Although the ratio of explicit to implicit socializing messages probably increases as children enter adolescence, implicit messages will always predominate. Thus, a more complete understanding of socialization at the intersection of race and math would need to incorporate observations of implicit socialization in the contexts of everyday life. Such observations would be well suited to capturing not only the subtleties of implicit socializing processes but also the subtleties of contemporary racial discrimination.

References

Boykin, A.W., & Toms, F.D. (1985). Black child socialization: A conceptual framework. In H.P. McAdoo & J.L. McAdoo (Eds.), *Black children: Social, environmental, and parental environments* (pp. 35–51). Newbury Park: Sage Publications.

Bracey, J.R. (2010). Socializing race: Parental beliefs and practices in two African *American families*. Unpublished doctoral dissertation, University of Illinois at Urbana-Champaign.

Burton, L.M., & Jarrett, R.L. (2000). In the mix, yet on the margins, the place of families in urban neighborhood and child development research. *Journal of Marriage and Family, 62*, 1114–1135.

Carter-Black, J. (2003). The myth of 'The tangle of pathology': Resilience strategies employed by middle-class African American families. *Journal of Family Social Work, 6*, 75–100.

Carter-Black, J. (2005). Success oriented strategies employed by middle-class African American families: A focus on positive racial identity development and socialization. (Doctoral dissertation). Retrieved from ProQuest Dissertations and Theses (UMI number 3202070).

Duncan, G.J., Huston, A.C., & Weisner, T.S. (2007). *Higher ground: New hope for the working poor and their children.* New York: Russell Sage.

Dyson, A.H. (2003). "Welcome to the jam": Popular culture, school literacy, and the making of childhoods. *Harvard Educational Review, 73*(3), 328–361.

Franklin, A.J., Boyd-Franklin, N., & Draper, C.V. (2002). A psychological and educational perspective on Black parenting. In H.P. McAdoo (Ed.), *Black children: Social, educational, and parental environments* (2nd ed., pp. 119–140). Thousand Oaks: Sage.

García Coll, C., & Marks, A.K. (2009). *Immigrant stories: Ethnicity and academics in middle childhood.* New York: Oxford University Press.

Hudley, E.P., Haight, W.L., & Miller, P.J. (2003). *'Raise up a child:' Human development in an African-American family.* Chicago: Lyceum.

Hughes, D., Rodriguez, J., Smith, E.P., Johnson, D.J., Stevenson, H.C., & Spicer, P. (2006). Parents' ethnic-racial socialization practices: A review of research and directions for future study. *Developmental Psychology, 42*, 747–770.

Jarrett, R. (2003). Worlds of development: The experiences of low-income, African American youth. *Journal of Children & Poverty, 9*, 157–189.

Mattison, E., & Aber, M.S. (2007). Closing the achievement gap: The association of racial climate with achievement and behavioral outcomes. *American Journal of Community Psychology, 40*, 1–12.

Miller, P.J., Cho, G.E., & Bracey, J. (2005). Working-class children's experience through the prism of personal storytelling. *Human Development, 48*, 115–135.

Miller, P.J., Fung, H., Lin, S., Chen, E.C., & Boldt, B.R. (2012). How socialization happens on the ground: Narrative practices as alternate socializing pathways in Taiwanese and European-American families. *Monographs of the Society for Research in Child Development*, 77(1), Serial No. 302.

Pattillo-McCoy, M. (1999). *Black picket fences: Privilege and peril among the Black middle class.* Chicago: The University of Chicago Press.

Slaughter-Defoe, D.T., Johnson, D.J., & Spencer, M.B. (2009). Race and children's development. In R.A. Shweder, T.R. Bidell, A.C. Dailey, S.D. Dixon, P.J. Miller & J. Modell (Eds.), *The child: An encyclopedic companion* (pp. 801–806). Chicago: The University of Chicago Press.

Steele, C.M., & Aronson, J. (1998). Stereotype threat and the test performance of academically successful African Americans. In C. Jencks & M. Phillips (Eds.), *The Black-White test score gap* (pp. 401–427). Washington: Brookings Institution.

Stevenson, H.C., McNeil, J.D., Herrero-Taylor, T., & Davis, G.Y. (2005). Influence of perceived neighborhood diversity and racism experience on the racial socialization of Black youth. *Journal of Black Psychology, 31*, 273–290.

Tatum, B.D. (1997). *'Why are all the Black kids sitting together in the cafeteria?'* New York: Basic Books.

Weisner, T.S., (Ed.). (2005). *Discovering successful pathways in children's development: Mixed methods in the study of childhood and family life.* Chicago: University of Chicago Press.

Dr. Peggy J. Miller (PhD 1979, Teachers College, Columbia University) is Professor Emerita in the Department of Psychology and the Department of Communication at the University of Illinois at Urbana-Champaign. She has published extensively on socialization through everyday narrative, with a focus on cultural and social class comparisons, and on ethnographic and qualitative methods. Her research is interdisciplinary, drawing on developmental psychology, cultural psychology, communication studies, and anthropology to craft a more culture-sensitive understanding of child development.

Dr. Jeana R. Bracey (PhD 2010, University of Illinois at Urbana-Champaign) is a Senior Associate at the Connecticut Center for Effective Practice of the Child Health and Development Institute of Connecticut. In addition to research on racial/ethnic socialization and identity development among children and youth, her professional interests include juvenile justice diversion, and program implementation and evaluation designed to improve program effectiveness and service delivery for youth with complex behavioral health needs and their families.

Peggy J. Miller
Department of Psychology
University of Illinois at Champaign-Urbana
603 East Daniel Street
Champaign-Urbana, IL 61820 (USA)
Tel. +1 217 344 6335, E-Mail pjm@illinois.edu

Commentary

Slaughter-Defoe DT (ed): Racial Stereotyping and Child Development.
Contrib Hum Dev. Basel, Karger, 2012, vol 25, pp 87–89

'What Does Race Have to Do with Math?' Relationships between Racial-Mathematical Socialization, Mathematical Identity, and Racial Identity

Commentary on English-Clarke, Slaughter-Defoe, and Martin

Margaret Beale Spencer

Department of Comparative Human Development, University of Chicago, Marshall Field IV Professor of Urban Education, Chicago, Ill., USA

During the previous half-century theorists have described the critical character of human competence and its linkages to psychosocial processes. Robert White's [1959, 1960] classic conceptualization of competence provides an excellent illustration of the process. His perspective suggests that individuals have a basic need to show agency. White hypothesizes that we are imbued with competence motivation and each possesses a basic interest in and need to demonstrate agency that is associated with and experienced affectively as a sense of competence. The general definition of competence suggests manifested effectiveness, successful task performance, or an ability to have an impact (i.e., to make a difference). Described over 50 years ago, White's [1959, 1960] competence motivation theoretical stance was not only useful in acknowledging the basic need for agency but successfully illustrated its affective parallel and described it as effectance/affectance motivation. The affective state accompanying manifested competence and general successes effectively demonstrate links between a particular experience or status having a social emotional correlate; competence formation processes suggest an internalization component leading to stable psychosocial processes. From a Phenomenological Variant of Ecological Systems Theory (PVEST) perspective (see fig. 1 in the paper by English-Clarke, Slaughter-Defoe, and Martin), White's definition illustrates why PVEST is necessarily a bi-directional and recursive framework [see Spencer, 1995, 2006].

The methodology utilized in the reported study and discussion of findings described by English-Clarke et al. appropriately illustrates that students' experiences with math concepts, as a potential challenge, can be both tracked back to parental socialization practices as well as linked, in forward fashion, to youths' subsequent identity processes. Equally important, PVEST serves as a helpful heuristic device since it is difficult to determine if parental socialization a priori serves primarily as a protective factor which affords youth with models of ego supports and confidence in the face of challenge or, recursively, if youths' manifested psychosocial processes and math performance and beliefs facilitate parental efforts through socialization strategies, thus, providing youth with models of adaptive coping responses.

The authors' use of the PVEST framework was appropriate, helpful and, in fact, assisted their explanations as to why future research, ideally utilizing both quantitative and qualitatively strategies, will be needed for an effective test of the hypotheses proposed. The strategy used in reporting the data provided an opportunity to examine the degree of agreement (or not) of youths' attitudes, perceptions and beliefs concerning mathematics with parental socialization efforts and math/racial identity processes. However, each component of the PVEST framework suggests *net* vulnerability level, stress engagement, reactive coping, and stable identity processes, thus, *both* positive and negative aspects of each of the components of PVEST were needed. That is, to effectively understand the net influence of the hypothesized socialization impact, both risks and protective factors needed to have been considered for understanding math competence or level of vulnerability. Further, it remains unclear whether or not more general parental math achievement socialization influences contributed to specific mathematics feedback as inferred or perceived by students.

Nonetheless the selection of PVEST as an organizing conceptual framework aided the valuable critique of the methodology employed, limitations of findings obtained, and possible explanations for the lack of definitiveness of hypothesized relationships. A more careful consideration of reactive coping processes such as youths' belief in the malleability or static character of intellectual functioning might also have assisted the interpretation of findings. Finally, future research that acknowledges the need to account for cumulative contributors due to the bidirectional and recursive influences of both risks and protective factors will aid the authors' ability to untangle the links of interest. In summary, the use of a theoretical perspective for framing the work is worthy of commendations in that it represents an important strength and conceptual innovation infrequently employed. In fact, the theoretical orientation incorporated for framing the project should serve the authors well as they continue work in this critically important line of education research.

References

Spencer, M.B. (1995). Old issues and new theorizing about African American youth: A phenomenological variant of ecological systems theory. In R.L. Taylor (Ed.), *Black youth: Perspectives on their status in the United States* (pp. 37–70). Westport, CT: Praeger.

Spencer, M.B. (2006). Phenomenology and ecological systems theory: Development of diverse groups. In W. Damon & R.M. Lerner (Series Eds.) & R.M. Lerner (Vol. Ed.), *Handbook of child psychology. Vol. I: Theoretical models of human development* (6th ed., pp. 829–893). Hoboken, NJ: Wiley.

White, R. (1959). Motivation reconsidered: The concept of competence. *Psychological Review, 66,* 297–333.

White, R. (1960). Competence and psychosexual development. In M.R. Riley (Ed.), *Nebraska symposium on motivation* (pp. 3–32). Lincoln: University of Nebraska Press.

Margaret Beale Spencer, PhD
University of Chicago, Marshall Field IV
Professor of Urban Education, Department of
Comparative Human Development
5730 South Woodlawn Avenue
Chicago, IL 60637 (USA)
Tel. +1 773 702 2496
E-Mail mbspencer@uchicago.edu

Dr. Margaret Beale Spencer (PhD 1976, University of Chicago) is the Marshall Field IV Professor of Urban Education in the Department of Comparative Human Development, and Professor in the Committee on Education and the College at the University of Chicago. Her theory-development scholarship focuses on child and adolescent resiliency, identity processes, and competence formation for ethnically diverse youth. Spencer has authored over 125 articles and chapters, has co-edited four volumes, is the recipient of funding from over three dozen federal and philanthropic agencies, and been the recipient of numerous honors and awards including elected (2009) membership into the National Academy of Education; a Society for Research in Child Development Distinguished Contribution Award; American Psychological Association (APA) Senior Career Award for Distinguished Contributions to Psychology in the Public Interest; Inaugural Fellow of AERA, and a Fletcher Fellowship recipient, which recognizes scholarship furthering the broad social goals of the US Supreme Court's Brown v. Board of Education Decision of 1954.

Paper

Slaughter-Defoe DT (ed): Racial Stereotyping and Child Development.
Contrib Hum Dev. Basel, Karger, 2012, vol 25, pp 90–104

On Researching the Agency of Africa's Young Citizens: Issues, Challenges and Prospects for Identity Development

A. Bame Nsamenang

University of Bamenda, Bamenda, Cameroon

Abstract

Over centuries, both scientific and popular literature on Africa's children has been generated mainly by the eclectic writings of Western travelers, merchants, missionaries, colonists, and lately by tourist researchers. Europeans engaged in Slave Trade in central and southern Africa between the fifteenth and eighteenth centuries noted that some children orphaned by famine sold their infant siblings for grain. Eurocentric literature on Africa is suffused with Darwinian insinuations and ethnocentrism, even racist ridicule. However, some also revealed that Africans understood children differently from Westerners, whose directive theories and narratives subvert Africa's ways of thinking about children and their development. This brief historical piece exposes three crucial lacunas, namely, the racism in child development science, the paucity of programmatic child development research, especially by African-born scholars, and the inattention to children's agency inherent in Africa's worldview and social capital. This chapter has sketched one framework for considering how to research some of the ways Africans, exemplified by Cameroonian parents, think about children and their development. It has overviewed the extent to which parental values permit and promote the agency by which children engage in self-learning and identity development within local peer cultures and global opportunities they co-construct.

Africa's ways of thinking about children and their development are somehow short chained into irrelevance and extinction by directive Western theories and narratives. Ever since imperialist ideologies and Social Darwinian motives penetrated Africa, Africa's knowledge increasingly ceased to be rooted in the African soil [Ojiaku, 1974]. Western theories and narratives censor African developmental knowledge and educational ideas, as conclusions on their research and analyses are progressively draped in Western theories and ideological perspectives. For instance, the few African scholars and policy developers who have the onerous task to research or plan African child development and education make a priori decisions within Western epistemologies and logic systems. They are forced by overly Western research and publication norms to address the universalizing Anglo-American image of childhood [Pence & Hix-Small, 2007; Prout & James, 1990] that drives the science of child development instead of analyzing, within cutting-edge scientific methodologies, the African children they experience in context as active and productive agents of their families and communities. They disappointingly persist in this intellectual mindset in spite of evidence from a Kenyan Gusii infant study that alternative patterns of care based on different moral and practical considerations can constitute normal patterns of development that had not been imagined in developmental theories [LeVine, 2004, p. 163].

This article is a thoroughly revised and extended update of a paper on child-to-child socialization in Cameroon I presented to the July 2010 International Society for the Scientific Study of Behavioral Development Conference in Lusaka, Zambia. It sketches one framework for understanding how to research some of the ways Africans in general and Cameroonian parents in particular think about their children and themselves within their worldviews and social capital. It specifically overviews the extent to which Africa's social capital and parental values permit and promote the agency by which children engage in self-education and orientate themselves in society and world through and within the cultural performances of familial and communal life and the social worlds they co-construct. This task is undertaken in seven parts. A brief methodological clarification follows this introductory piece and precedes a theoretic orientation. The fourth section is devoted to archival evidence of agency in African children, with illustrative examples from the parenting and peer cultures of the author's home turf, Cameroon, articulated within the extant literature. The fifth part endeavors to make explicit how a sense of agency connects with self-construal and identity development in Africa's young citizens. The sixth part is a discussion that muses over the implications and fate of children's agency vis-à-vis a clearly Euro-American science of child development. The chapter concludes by refocusing on African children as competent participants in cultural communities.

Method

Triangulated Archival Evidence
This paper is theoretical but framed on triangulated archival evidence from the author's research and selected English language sources available to the author. Initial impressions were obtained from a 1989 extensive survey of cohorts of Nso parents about their values for children and care of a targeted child [see Nsamenang, 1992a; Nsamenang & Lamb, 1993, 1994, 1995].

A second source of evidence comes from a 1991 weeklong observation study of the social ecology of rural and urban Nso infants in northwest Cameroon. Observations were made in Nso villages (rural sample) and an urban sample was observed in Nso settler population in Bamenda 110 km away from Nso homeland [Nsamenang, 1991]. The focal themes of the observation were the physical organization of the home, infant spaces, caregiving routines, primary caregivers, responsibility sharing, sleeping patterns, infant social settings, including visiting adults and accompanying infants, among other facets of infant ecology.

The third source includes work in local development and global networks (e.g., Nsamenang [2002, 2004, 2006], Dasen [1984], Dasen, Inhelder, Lavallee & Retschitzi [1978], Erny [1968, 1973, 1987], Rabain [1979], Rabain-Jamin [2003], Jahoda [1982], Serpell [1993, 1994], Harkness & Super [1992], and Zimba [2002]).

Theoretic Moorings
Human sages have claimed a distinct identity for their species. In the animal kingdom the human being is the only animal that is alleged to experience its own existence. Thus, the notion of self implies a sense of reflective self-awareness, with self-perception being a significant marker of self-construal in the process of identity development [Smith, Bond & Kağitçibaşi, 2006]. I am using 'self' here as a social product that emerges out of social interaction and is socially situated in time and context [Kağitçibaşi, 2007]. It is honed by an emergent self-awareness.

The concept of children's agency has been used in varied ways; this chapter examines children as cognizing and experiencing 'agents' who are capable of autonomous action and cultural creation [Nsamenang, 2008]. Agency is a theoretic concept that positions children as self-conscious members of the family and society right from the beginning. Children are active participants in family and communal life. There is no doubt that children are agentive in the sense of having the capacity to experience, make meaning, interact, act, produce and reproduce progressively in the course of development. For example, lack of commercial toys prompts most African children to create their own playthings from local materials [Nsamenang & Lamb, 1994]. Furthermore, adult male labor migration throughout Africa emboldened boys and girls to acquaint themselves with new cultural possibilities and economic conduits through which they accumulate and build up their own resources to accelerate their own ascent to seniority [Richards, 1996].

In the socialization literature, the parent, particularly the mother, almost universally has been presented as the primary source of a child's nurturance and developmental knowledge during the early years [e.g., Bossard & Boll, 1966; Lerner, 2002]. Sub-Saharan African cultures understand the role of a child differently from their Western counterparts, especially the evolution of the elite monogamous parents depicted by Ariès [1962]. Africa's worldview and developmental ethos bracket chronological age on social competence in tacit alertness to the potential and sometimes experienced incongruence between biological age and social competence [Nsamenang, 1992a, 2004, 2006]. African cultures separate the learning of skills for socially shared support of the family [Weisner, 1987] from the life stage of parenthood but integrate them into cultural curricula for children to learn as part of their developmental knowledge [Nsamenang, 2008]. From their toddler years, even from younger ages, most African children are immersed in social networks in homes, schools, and diverse neighborhood settings in which parents or other adults only partially play direct developmental roles or inputs, as siblings or peers become more salient developmental partners in children's daily routines.

In contrast, dominant Western developmental theories position caregiving as a specialized task of adulthood and distance children away from it in educational institutions and non-adult play spheres. Nonetheless, even in the West there is evidence that age does not always match with functional ability, as younger (more intelligent) children have succeeded in tasks on which older sibs or peers have faltered. Solberg [1995], a Norwegian sociologist, coined the term *social age* to refer to negotiated conceptions of being older or younger, a more flexible construct than chronological age. Solberg's [1995] research revealed that ten-year-old children and their employed mothers held quite different views on children taking care of themselves at home after school. The mothers worried that their children returned home to an 'empty house,' but some of the children spoke instead of coming home to a 'welcoming house' with independent access to household facilities that would be impossible in the presence of parents.

Africa's developmental trajectories are symbolized in garden metaphors such as seeding, cultivation and fruit bearing. The seeds are typically nurtured or cultivated into maturity not in gardens of monoculture to highlight lonesome individualism but in polycultures that underline intersubjective individuation [Nsamenang, 2004]. Garden metaphors suggest gradual unfolding of developmental abilities and serialized attainment of levels of maturity and culturally valued skills and competencies at various 'stations' of social ontogeny. Devor's [1970] interpretation of agent as shorthand for *agent of socialization* fits with African theories that exude parental values that recognize children's innate abilities for reciprocal socialization, collective learning and peer mentoring [Nsamenang, 2002, 2004]. Inducted into such theories, with supportive social capital, African parents socialize children in the children's *becoming* [Erny, 1968], 'not as a set of organisms to be molded into a pattern of behavior specified in advance as educational outcomes, but as newcomers to a community of practice, for whom the desirable outcome of a period of apprenticeship is that they would appropriate the system of meanings that informs the community's practices' [Serpell, 2008, p. 74].

Within the theoretic framework of agency, children should neither be analyzed as outsiders to society nor as mere inductees into adult society; rather, they are bona fide citizens with interests, talents, collaborative actions and resistances (Convention on the Rights of the Child 1989 [see UNICEF, 2003]) and their collective action must therefore be taken into explicit account in theory, research and policy. Within the framework of Hart's [2002] wisdom, agency calls for science-based proliferation of strategies to ease Africa's young citizens' reflective appraisals of their appalling conditions so that they would begin to gradually take greater responsibility as they develop for creating societies and nations different from the ones they live in or have inherited.

Developmental Agency within Africa's Social Capital and Parental Values

Developmental learning refers to knowledge and skills acquisition that is vital to children's survival and development, which children do not possess at birth [Nsamenang, 2011a] but that they can learn, sometimes without the usual notion of schools and classrooms [Bruner, 1996]. This genre of learning is an African reality that neither trivializes nor queries the indispensability of school learning. Nevertheless, this viewpoint challenges the conjecture that without schools or academic pipelines [Cooper & Gandara, 2001] children cannot learn and alludes to viable but unexplored nonacademic pathways outside the school system in Africa for investigative discovery and enhancement [Nsamenang, 2011a]. We need to focus research attention on the agentive strategies with which African children navigate the harsh realities of their circumstances to survive and make progress on their own devices! The evidence for such agency is more evident within African family traditions and peer cultures than in the school or formal institutional education, though versions of it are to be found therein; they remain mostly unexploited, however. The largely ignored ingenuities that underwrite indigenous African craft and art work have their origins in such inventive agency, but spuriously adopted colonial school curricula, research agendas and policy development in much of Africa have hitherto ignored its potentially transformative processes and outcomes.

A holistic and non-Cartesian African cosmology interconnects the sacred and the secular worlds and visualizes them as conceptually inseparable [Bongmba, 2001]. African theories of the universe situate the child as a cultural agent who must undertake a cultural curriculum at various stages of development. The family is central to this role; because it is the institutional hub in which childbearing and childrearing are located, such that childcare is a collective enterprise rather than a parental prerogative [Nsamenang, 1992a]. In the southern Africa region, an indigenous social support network is reserved for newborns and their mothers [Zimba, 2002, p. 94]. In Eastern and Western Africa, newborns are treated like 'precious treasures' that are nurtured by the whole family [Harkness & Super, 1992] in a deep and comforting sense of tradition and community [Nsamenang, 1992b]. The Western child development literature aptly places the primary duty for young children's social security and care on mothers, but analysis of traditional childcare in Africa would reveal a landscape in which African mothers are partially available, enacting the supervisor role, while the bulk of the day care and social security of children after they have been weaned reverts to older siblings and their peer group [Nsamenang, 1992b].

African families permit and guide the social and cognitive transformation of children through child work, which is an indispensable mode of preparing the next generation. Planned in synergy, it can complement rather than subvert school learning. The family and the child understand it as useful to the family and necessary for the child's developmental learning and social integration. It is graduated on the culture's perceived developmental trajectory and the child's level of developmental competence. Through it, children become independent at an early age, and this independence is fostered and enforced by letting a child do even difficult things on his own [Munday, 1979, p. 165]. Social and intellectual transformation in the child is brought about by participation in family and societal life [Rogoff, 2003]. African families do not traditionally tolerate child abuse through work that is not the participative mode of education and civic sensitization [Nsamenang, 1992a]. However, participatory learning is open to abuse and, indeed, has been abused by individuals and families. The confusion between child work and child abuse is only one of several issues that complicate the study and intervention on behalf of African children.

Children in Africa perform a much wider range of caring roles and socially and economically productive activities than is the case in most other societies. Children take on real family duties such as sibling caregiving [Chiakem, 2009], household chores [Nsamenang, 1992a, b], and running errands [Ogunaike & Houser, 2002]. Parents scaffold the responsibilities they assign to children according to children's perceived maturity and capability. From an early age, children are allowed to observe and gradually participate in family tasks and caregiving to younger sibs, each according to demonstrated developmental ability or competence [Nsamenang, 1992b; Weisner, 1987]. Thus, children's agency entails hands-on processes that invoke dependence, interdependence, vulnerability, need, and development, all of which should come into research focus. This should not just be in the study of children but also adults, since these issues are also evident in adult experiences. The Africentric sense of agentive engagement calls for research that seeks to clarify how to situate and enhance Africa's next generations – children and youth – as the continent's fragile bridge into an uncertain globalized future.

Given the high density of children per African family, as evidenced by 4.7 siblings in the Bamenda Grassfields of Cameroon [Nsamenang, 1992a] and a West African range of 4.5 in Cameroon to 7.0 siblings in Ivory Coast [Ware, 1983], toddlers in Africa are more likely to experience daytime interaction with peers or siblings rather than with 'busy' mothers or other adults [Ogbimi & Alao, 1998]. The social world of African childhoods

typically is a multi-aged, mixed-ability, interactive context that contrasts with that of the dyadic microsystem of parent-child, child-teacher, and practitioner-child that has gained analytical force in childhood research [Nsamenang, 2010]. A typical daytime neighborhood scenario is a 'gang' of multi-age, mixed-sex children with one or two 10- to 12-year-old preadolescents as their protective supervisors [Nsamenang, 1992b]. Evidence from research with Nso children [e.g., Nsamenang, 2011a] and archival sources from across Africa is adding to knowledge of children's 'developmental emergence' into adolescence and adulthood as actors in their own right although their contribution to their developmental learning is yet to gain acceptable entry into the discipline's knowledge base. The bulk of such contributions occurs primarily in social exchanges and distributive norms of different social sectors and activity settings in which the young engage with significant others such as parents, adult caregivers, teachers, and peers. As children develop, they gradually and systematically enter into and assume different levels of personhood, identity, and being; they 'graduate' from one role setting and participative sphere to another, until they transition gradually into adulthood. Boys and girls emerging into adulthood are best evaluated for proficiency in sibling and peer cultures rather than in adult-child spaces [Nsamenang, 2010].

African children's agency is discernible in parental values that permit peer group life and support self-care and performance of household duties from an early age. It is also noticeable in children's capacity to transcend adult models by creating their own social worlds, even when living up to adult orders [Nsamenang & Lamb, 1995]. Children's agency and protagonism is also evident in young carers who support ailing parents or ageing guardians, especially those affected by HIV/AIDS. Drawing on data collected in Western Kenya, Skovdal, Ogutu, Aoro & Campbell [2009] reported how young carers coped with challenging circumstances, often with skill and ingenuity. They concluded that children's ability to cope with adversity was determined by the extent of their community participation and proficiency in negotiating for social and material support from it. Their data revealed how young carers mobilized social support, engaged in income generating activities, and constructed positive social identities around their caring roles.

Self-Construal and Identity Development: A Multifaceted, Context-Sensitive Process

Self-development or individuation is the process through which the child systematically defines and distills the 'self' from the 'non-self'. Individuation theoretically sets an individual apart from social others; through it a child increasingly defines who she/he is by differentiating the self (that which is me) from the non-self (that which is not me) during different phases of life. Defining the self or spelling out who one is in relation to and interaction with social others is an essential developmental task in three components. First, a personal factor involves an ongoing seeking and clarifying 'who am I' as the one and only *individuum*, distinct from the non-self. The second component is group-specific and depends on group mission and mores, say, a peer group, youth gang, study group, religious sect, and degree of fidelity to its norms. Third, a cultural facet that derives from what personhood within one's ethnic or racial community and current social and developmental status within its norms is and normatively entails [see Nsamenang, 2011a, p. 247]. During individuation into hierarchical social networks and relationships with others, the child increasingly defines and sharpens these facets of selfhood. Self-concept and agency add to nature and nurture as a third developmental force [Nsamenang, 2005], implying that sense of direction, cognition and deliberate pursuit of personal goals channel development. Indeed, self-concept is a self-conscious agentive force that impels developmental outcomes [Nsamenang, 2008].

The preceding section depicted the developmental context of the African child as a mixed sociological garden wherein adults and children share roles in nurturing the child and performing livelihood chores. The metaphor for identity development in this social garden is polycropping, not monoculture, because the emphasis on self-construal and identity formation is on the shared and social rather than the unique and individual aspects of personhood. African parents sensitize children from an early age to seek out others from whom to extract local knowledge and situated 'intelligences' and in so doing clarify who they are, particularly within sibling and peer spaces. Children extort the social, emotional, practical, cognitive, relational values and other norms ingrained in the activity settings of the home, society, and peer cultures more through their contextual embedment and active participation and less through explicit adult instruction. In so doing they 'graduate' from one activity setting and participative sector of the peer culture to another, steadily maturing toward adult identity and roles. The 'extractive' processes they engage are similar to the interactional-extractive learning process Piaget [1952] invoked, but differ in being child-to-child interstimulation and mentorship. That is, the mentors in most children's zone of proximal development [Vygotsky, 1978] are not adults but siblings and peers, who initiate and promote considerable self-education and developmental gains from and through cooperation and antagonism with others. Zimba [2002, p. 94] described one instance of self-definition with the Zulu community of South Africa, as nurturing *umuntu umuntu ngabantu*, which literally translates into 'a person is only a person with other people'. This relational view of identity development downplays sovereign individuation, implying that a sense of self cannot be attained or adequately understood without reference to the 'community' of other humans.

By positioning children as emerging into levels of selfhood, implying the unfolding of biological potentialities and social competencies, Africans tacitly acknowledge that self-concept evolves with a maturing self-consciousness that accords a sense of self-direction and agentive search for or choice of the resources and exposures that increasingly differentiate and polish self-identity and goal-directed behavior toward desired or imagined personal status, either of sovereign individuality or relational individuality [Kağitçibaşi, 2007; Nsamenang, 2004]. Such a dynamic developmental perspective affirms the view that legal identity is established from birth, whereas personal, social, and cultural identity grows and changes [Woodhead, 2008, p. 4]. In a nutshell, the process of developing a sense of self is a process of connecting individual personal identity to a changing social identity, depending on a child's ontogenetic group affiliations [Pence & Nsamenang, 2008, p. 41].

Individualism and connectedness are not dichotomous human qualities; they develop together in the same child. The child therefore individuates or evolves a self-identity by being systematically socialized and educated, if not indoctrinated, into being interconnected to or detached from social others. What accounts for relational or independent self-construal may not be inborn in individuals, but is socially scripted or constructed and nudged unobtrusively into childrearing regimes and educational traditions, for example, cultural scripts of family-based social capital and mutual reciprocity versus those of centrally organized social security provisioning and purchasable social security services. Because children are initially dependent, they follow an interconnected or aloof self-construal in conformity to the norms of their culture and social networks, particularly those of familial, religious, and peer group networks. Accordingly, selfhood or individuality becomes meaningful primarily in the light of a child's social networks, although universal facets of individuality may traverse social turfs.

The interdependent or relational identities of Africans do not at all obliterate their individuality. Individualism-collectivism research has hitherto focused mostly on the cultural (external) component of African children's identity. An important theoretical concern and methodological issue pertains to why research on collectivism-individualism with African children has not addressed the psychic or inner attributes inherent in African individuation processes [Nsamenang, 2004, p. 118]. This shortsightedness is the more surprising given theorists' and scholars' awareness that learning actively engages individualized cognitive repertoires and that development itself is an interiorized process by which the child, like the adult, autonomously exercises cognitive and personal abilities or perceived contextual inputs. Children and youth elaborate and organize their capacities to achieve learning outcomes or developmental changes. This provokes the seemingly trite but so far mutedly significant theoretic issue that no one else can actually learn or develop for another.

Individuation or child development occurs neither in a vacuum nor in a universal civilization. Across cultures and contexts, it unfolds within the potentials set by an individualized genotype and the facilitating or constraining forces of diverse cultural curricula. While heredity prewires development, cultural tools and nurturing regimes supply the 'content' that accords meaning and sense of direction to self-construal and identity development. Culture may be external to individuals but its expression emerges from individual 'skins', teased out by specific contextual factors [Nsamenang, 2011a]. Culture, as in social heritage and cultural artifacts and tools, complements genotype to shape individuation and psychosocial differentiation in the direction of given children's cultural meaning systems [Nsamenang, 2008, p. 213]. This implies that context and culture complement personalized genotypes to shove developmental trajectories and psychosocial differentiation and identity development in this and not that direction, therein creating and magnifying diversity in phenotypes or individualities. By fostering children's close identification with social networks and peer contexts, African social values can be seen to align with Erikson's [1968] focus on social development. For example, African social rites of naming, marriage, death, etc. effortlessly transition the identity of the individual through developmental phases [Pence & Nsamenang, 2008].

The developmental nature of identity formation invokes issues of stability in personal and group identity. Part of identity includes a sense of continuity and group affiliation – a social identity. Individuals gain a personal identity and social identity by their affiliation to various groups – family, peer groups, racial group, ethnic culture, and national community. Many social scientists regard ethnic or racial identity, that is, the enduring, fundamental aspect of the self that includes a subjective sense of membership in an ethnic or racial group, to be one of the many facets of an individual's social identity with important real world implications for intergroup relations [Phinney & Baldelomar, 2011]. Cultural identity is the identity felt by being a member of a group or culture, or of an individual as far as influenced by her/his belonging to a cultural or ethnic group. The development of ethnic identity is determined by what the majority of adults in a given society at a particular historical point consider to be prominent and acceptable or valuable and functional. Group affiliation and collective identity help people define themselves in the eyes of others and themselves [Sall & Nsamenang, 2011].

Societies have histories in the course of which identities emerged or weakened; specific historical structures engender identity types that become recognizable in individualized profiles. Recognition by others as a distinct ethnic or racial group is often a contributing factor to developing or resisting a social identity. Ethnic groups are also often united by common cultural, behavioral, linguistic, ritualistic, or religious traits, the so-called behavioral tendencies. National identity is a philosophical concept that assigns all humans to groups called nations. Members of a nation are expected to share a common identity, and usually a common origin, in the sense of ancestry, parentage or descent. But most nation states in Africa were not constituted on this basis; they were carved out by arbitrary state boundaries sequel to European partition of Africa at the 1884 Berlin Congress, a political surgery that split many African ethnic identities into two or more colonies and, later, into independent successor states [Asiwaju, 1984]. Centuries of Slave Trade forced hundreds of ethnic African youth into a journey of no return into the Americas, a significant portion of them being American citizens who identify today as African-Americans.

Identity formation has been most extensively described by Erikson [1968], who saw identity formation as beginning in childhood and gaining prominence during adolescence. Faced with physical growth, sexual maturation, and impending career choices and family formation, adolescents must accomplish the task of integrating their prior experiences and characteristics into a stable adult identity. Erikson coined the phrase 'identity crisis' to describe the temporary instability and confusion adolescents experience as they struggle with competing alternatives and choice points. In Africa today, confusion and crises are inherent in old and new ways coexisting in the same countries, communities, and individual lives [Nsamenang & Dawes, 1998]. Africans have become purveyors and peddlers of foreign ideas, tastes, lifestyles, and cultural fragments that are largely at variance with 'the soil out of which the existing African society has grown and the human values it has produced' [Kishani, 2001, p. 37]. Imagine, for example, that in African family traditions children are accredited participants in agrarian life but that school learning rids Africa's children of their farming skills!

The net outcome of the foregoing is that most African young citizens (and growing numbers of professionals) only visualize their fate and future outside of their homelands, albeit in precarious immigration conditions in recipient countries.

Thus, a recent study in Cameroon [Nsamenang, 2011b] recorded almost unanimous youth endorsement of immigration to Europe. Their personal confusion and identity crisis deepen with the emergence of views that are similar to that of one adolescent respondent: '... this corrupt country is without opportunities; I study and this is apparently an advantage, but I can't expect anything; the only clear possibility I have is to continue studying and try to get out of the country as soon an opportunity offers; here, there is no future' (author's translation) [Nsamenang, 2011b, pp. 153–154]. Nevertheless, the majority of African children and youth are not overly defeated by their difficult circumstances but instead navigate their challenges successfully into productive pathways, surprisingly often outside official agendas. More research is needed about how these African youth successfully produce competent African self-identities.

Discussion

Implications for Scientific Research and Social Science Policies for African Children Research
Decades ago, Schildkrout [1978] noted the underrepresentation of children in descriptions of social systems. Children, particularly African children, are still sparsely represented in research and social discourse reflective of their huge numbers and significance as the *root of humanity* [Lanyasunya & Lesolayia, 2001]. Schildkrout [1978] proposed that children should be understood as children rather than as the next generation of adults. Reversing the familiar equation of children as non-adults [Munday, 1979], Schildkrout [1978] aptly asked, 'What would happen to the adult world (other than its extinction) if there were no children?' and 'In what ways are adults dependent upon children?' Drawing upon fieldwork with the Hausa, a Muslim society in Nigeria, Schildkrout [1974] described children's contributions to sustaining the religious institution of purdah that involves the spatial seclusion of women. Among the Hausa, married men earn income away from their households as butchers and artisans; women earn money by cooking food and embroidering assorted wares to sell at local markets. Confined to their households by purdah, income-earning women depend on children to purchase materials and to deliver and sell their products at the market. Up until puberty, both girls and boys are free to move between markets and households. These Nigerian Hausa arrangements, common in most Muslim communities, with spatially mobile prepubescent boys and girls actively contributing to economic and religious institutions, reverse late-twentieth-century Western assumptions about children's place and highlight varied constructions of both childhood and adulthood. Such contributions by networks of children to social, economic and religious life persist throughout Africa today, alongside the newly imported versions that are given priority research and policy attention for enhancement interventions.

The active but tacit principle in children's contributions is 'better together' [Rogoff, Turkanis, & Bartlett, 2000], as these contributions support their social cognition and social development. 'Social cognition' means being able to understand our own and others' thoughts, desires, intentions, and feelings [CEECD, 2011]. Children begin to develop social skills when they understand how people's thoughts, desires, intentions, and feelings affect the way they act and behave. Interaction in mixed-age groups elicits prosocial behaviors and social cognition that are important in the social and cognitive development of the young child. Such prosocial behaviors as help-giving, sharing, and turn-taking facilitate interaction and promote socialization and affective bonding. Thus, peer cultures are childhood spaces for socializing, exploratory play, play and learning, differing and worrying in child-to-child worlds with limited to no adult presence. More importantly, peer cultures train in responsibility taking, but lamentably, African peer spaces have been little researched and remain uncharted developmental niches.

Multi-age, multi-sex peer groups offer greater freedom to children to function on their own terms than adult-child relationships. In them, children learn from competition, cooperation, antagonisms and handling of conflicts and problems with minimal to no adult intrusion. The prime advantage of mixed age groups is that children learn from each other – younger from older, and older from younger. Older children learn to adapt their language and social skills to relate with younger children, often learning patience, compassion, perspective-taking and problem solving skills. Younger children are challenged by older sibs and peers to engage in more complex activities than when they are with their parents or other adults. Children create and maintain cultural environments which are appropriate for themselves [Rabain-Jamin, 2003] and adopt as well as re-invent their own language [Ochs, 1988]. Responsible intelligence [Nsamenang, 2006] inheres in peer group activities, particularly in the extensive child-to-child sociability in the different activity sectors and spheres and in the real family duties children perform, as the welfare of the family would be at risk if they fail in task performance. It thus seems plausible to chart the social learning and cognitive values and abilities inherent in 'child work'.

Social perceptions among peers play a key role in the development of social competence and cognitive abilities. They are an essential part of a child's increasing social awareness, sociability and cognitive repertoire. The formation of friendships is often based on a child's perceptions of the differing roles of peers in a variety of interactive contexts. Research evidence [e.g., CEECD, 2011] suggests that children of different ages are usually aware of differences and attributes associated with age. As they mature, children become able to cognize what they and other people cherish, want, think or know. They also understand that people express different emotions depending on

situation (example: knowing that an individual is happy when she gets what she wants or sad if he does not). As a result, both younger and older children in mixed-age groups differentiate their expectations depending on the ages of the participants. In fact, once children join the peer group, they begin to carve out their own sub-niches in terms of identifying secure and reliable others who support them and from whom they abstract the norms and ways of the world and a sense of security [Nsamenang, 2002].

If prosocial behaviors are indices of social development and social cognition, then, we need to document those that are more tacit than explicit in African developmental processes in general and children's agency in particular. William Corsaro [1990] observed preschoolers in the United States and in Italy and recorded how they created distinctive peer cultures from their use of ideas from the adult world. Similarly, Nsamenang and Lamb [1995] referred to Nso children as not being passive followers of adult values and norms but as creative producers of their own social worlds. Corsaro [1990] coined the term *interpretive reproduction* to explain children's cultural production and introduction of change. On his part, Vygotsky [1978] believed that the internalization of children's new understandings or 'cognitive restructuring' occurs when concepts are actually transformed and not merely replicated. He [Vygotsky, 1978, p. 86] asserted that internalization takes place when children interact within their 'zone of proximal development' (ZPD) which he defined as the distance between the actual development level of a child as determined by independent problem solving and the level of potential development as determined through problem solving under adult guidance. African theories prime individuation and promote cooperative intellectual development in a Vygotskian sense, but whereas the adult plays a pivotal role in Vygotsky's [1978] ZPD, the African ZPD is largely learning in child-to-child sociability and mentorship [Nsamenang, 2008].

Slavin [1987] suggests that in terms of the Vygotskian concept of ZPD, the discrepancy between what a child can do with and without assistance can be the basis for cooperative peer efforts that result in cognitive gains. Slavin [1987] views collaborative activity among children as promoting growth because children of similar ages are likely to be operating within one another's zones of proximal development, modeling in the collaborating group behaviors more advanced than those they could perform as individuals. Brown and Reeve [1985] maintain that instruction aimed at a wide range of abilities allows the novice to learn at his own rate and to manage various cognitive challenges in the presence of peer 'experts'. One source of impact of mixed-age grouping on cognition is assumed to be the disputes and conflicts that arise from children's interaction with peers of different levels of cognitive maturity. In their discussion of cognitive conflict, Brown and Palinscar [1985] make the point that the contribution of cognitive conflicts to learning is not simply that the less-informed child *imitates* the more knowledgeable one. The interaction and interstimulation between the children lead the novice child to *internalize* new understandings.

Childhood Science and Social Policy
Children and childhood are discursively constructed not only by scholars and the media, but also by corporations that design and sell goods to expanding child and youth markets [Steinberg & Kincheloe, 2004]. Childhood is a social construct [Jenks, 1982, p. 12] wherein all cultures recognize, define and assign different cultural curricula and developmental tasks to the same maturing human biology [Nsamenang, 1992, p. 144]. If child development is a universal phenomenon that unfolds from an individualized genotype in context-sensitive and culture-imbued transactional processes, then research, theory, and policy, defined inclusively, must integrate the variety of childhoods [Prout & James, 1990, p. 12] that exists across cultures rather than persist with a single,

Western-crafted image of children that is increasingly becoming standardized [Pence & Hix-Small, 2007]. In this sense, the dominance of child development science by Euro-American values, theories and narratives is insulting as it presents only a lopsided picture of the childhoods that should be the science's principal task to equitably explore and document.

Alleged state-of-the-art child development texts are suffused with Western childhood realities and ideological values [Zornado, 2001]. Howitt and Owusu-Bempah [1994] interpreted the racism in the contents and organization of psychology textbooks and institutions, as 'a broad assault on the nature of black cultures' (p. 71). Opportunely, most gate keepers of the field 'are keenly aware that research based on a predominantly Western scientific paradigm is part of the story, but not the full story needed to move forward' the field, especially in local development [Arnold, 2004, p. 46]. Yet, the science continues to circumvent the childhoods of 95% of the world's population living in the Majority (nonwestern) World, tending to dismiss them as antiprogressive, while relying on American Psychology producing 'research findings that implicitly apply to the entire human population, the entire species' [Arnett, 2008, p. 602].

A global watchdog – the United Nations – is staffed with some of the best experts who are clearly aware that the developmentally appropriate practices they apply present only an appearance of science-based knowledge in formulas framed heavily by Western cultural ideologies [LeVine, 2004]. Rights-based thinking and global age emphases on the belief that 'all cultures can contribute scientific knowledge of universal value' [UNESCO, 1999] should oblige the United Nations, its multiple agencies, gate keepers of scientific disciplines, and those who work in international development to feel edgy about the imperious tinge of the knowledge systems and frameworks with and within which they address global issues and craft international child development instruments and policy guidelines. The UNCRC (United Nations Convention on the Rights of the Child), for example, has been justifiably criticized for having been 'developed far from the lived experience of children, their families and communities' [Reid, 2006, p. 18].

In *From innocents to agents: Children and children's rights in New Zealand*, Reid [2006] further differentiated between advocates and parents, pointing to how growing networks of powerful advocacy agencies have caged parents and 'captured' children's rights, intensifying the ambiguity as to who holds the primary rights for children. The net impact of Africa relying in the long-term on Western norms is suppression of local developmental knowledge and practices, therein denying equity and emasculating African children's cultural identities in transgression of the Convention on the Rights of the Child [CRC, UNICEF, 2003] that enshrines rights to a cultural identity.

Conclusion

As childhood is entering the central agendas of African governments [Pence & Marfo, 2008], Africans, like the global community, are being alerted to how participation furthers children's survival, protection, and development, and how children as rights-bearers can contribute and bring change to society [Cook, Blanchet-Cohen & Hart, 2004]. The CRC acclaims children's place in civil society as partners with other social players and proposes a major shift in the social representation of children, who should no longer be defined as 'problems' or 'victims' but as active social agents. Views of children as adults-in-the-making minimize their citizenship status as rights-holders who deserve being studied in their own right as full social actors instead of being framed in research and programs as emerging adults who add to problems for the adult social order. This means that children have rights and are judged capable of striving to achieve these rights if they are denied

or violated. Yet, the protagonism of the bulk of Africa's active population – children and youth – has been condemned as child abuse by international advocacy and child-rights activists.

Sadly, various forms of child labor, child abuse, even child enslavement, are increasingly and condemnably sneaking into Africa's developmental task of child work. However, these undesirable forms are what ought to be criminalized and extinguished, *not* the hands-on responsibility-training component of Africa's family-based education that requires research-based understanding and enhancement, and that should be integrated into school curricula and early childhood development programs.

Scrutiny of mainstream developmental science literature would generate an image of children and adolescents as non-adults [Munday, 1979] lacking the maturity and agency to act sensibly on their own self-interest. By contrast, African theories and social capital permit and foster children's active agency in self-education [Pence & Nsamenang, 2008]. The search for contextually receptive and culturally suitable strategies to actualize the CRC provisions on children's citizenship and participation is emerging but also confusing. If researchers could listen to Africa, the science could gain from Africa's holistic view of the child as integrated in a context [Callaghan, 1989]. In so doing, we must critically analyze concerns that 'in Britain too little is expected of children, their activities being restricted almost entirely to play' [Ellis, 1978, p. 50] and why American children whose developmentally appropriate norms are proselytized to the rest of the world are said to be 'underemployed' [Zelizer, 1985, p. 208]. If we could conceptualize children as competent *participants in cultural communities* [Rogoff, 2003], we would avoid such unease because contextualist research would outsource strategies that reach out to children in their contexts and that permit community ownership and participation.

References

Aries, P. (1962). *Centuries of childhood: A social history of family life.* Translated by Robert Baldick. New York: Knopf.

Arnett, J.J. (2008). The neglected 95%: Why American psychology needs to become less American. *American Psychologist, 63,* 602–614.

Arnold, C. (2004). Positioning ECCD in the 21st century. *Coordinators' Notebook, 28,* 1–36.

Asiwaju, A.I. (1984). Partitioned Africa: Ethnic relations across Africa's international borders, 1884–1984. Lagos, Nigeria: University of Lagos Press.

Bongmba, E.K. (2001). *African witchcraft and otherness: A philosophical and theological critique of intersubjective relations.* New York: New York University Press.

Bossard, J.H., & Bell, E.S. (1966). *The sociology of the child.* New York: Harper & Row.

Brown, A.L., & Reeve, R.A. (1985). *Bandwidths of competence: The role of supportive contexts in learning and development* (Technical Rep. No. 336). Champaign: Centre for the Study of Reading.

Brown, A.L., & Palinscar, A. (1986). *Guided cooperative learning and individual knowledge acquisition* (Technical Rep. No. 372). Champaign: Centre for the Study of Reading.

Bruner, J. (1996). *The culture of education.* Cambridge: Harvard University Press.

Callaghan, L. (1998). Building on an African worldview. *Early Childhood Matters, 89,* 30–33.

CEECD (Centre of Excellence for Early Childhood Development) (2011). *Social cognition: Helping your child understand people's thoughts and feelings.* Montreal: GRIP-Université de Montréal.

Chiakem, O. (2009). *The role of sibling caretakers in the development of social abilities in younger children.* A Master of Education Dissertation, Department of Educational Psychology, Faculty of Education, University of Buea, Cameroon.

Cook, P., Blanchet-Cohen, N., & Hart, S. (2004). *Children as partners: Child participation in promoting social change.* Victoria: IICRD.

Cooper, C., & Gandara, P. (2001). Guest Editors' introduction: When diversity works: Bridging families, peers, schools and communities at CREDE. *Journal of Education for Students Placed at Risk, 6,* i–iv.

Corsaro, W.A. (1990). The underlife of nursery school: Young children's social representations of adult roles. In G. Duven & B. Lloyd (Eds.), *Social participation and the development of knowledge.* Cambridge: Cambridge University Press.

Dasen, P.R. (1984). The cross-cultural study of intelligence: Piaget and the Baoule. *International Journal of Behavioral Development, 19,* 407–434.

Dasen, P.R., Inhelder, R., Lavallee, M., & Retschitzi, J. (1978). *Naissance de l'intelligence chez l'enfant Baoule de Cote d'Ivoire.* Berne: Hans Huber.

Devor, G.M. (1970). Children as agents of socializing parents. *The Family Coordinator, 19,* 208–212.

Ellis, J. (1978). *West African families in Great Britain.* London: Routledge.

Erikson, E. (1968). *Childhood and society.* Harmondsworth: Penguin.

Erny, P. (1968). *L'Enfant dans la pensée traditionnelle d'Afrique Noire.* Paris: Le Livre Africain.

Erny, P. (1973). *Childhood and cosmos: the social psychology of the Black African child.* New York: New Perspectives.

Erny, P. (1987). *L'enfant et son milieu Afrique Noire.* Paris: L'Harmattan.

Harkness, S., & Super, C.M. (1992). Shared childcare in East Africa: Socio-cultural origins and developmental consequences. In M.E. Lamb, K.J. Sternberg, C.P. Hwang & A.G. Broberg (Eds.), *Child care in context: Socio-cultural perspectives* (pp. 441–459). Hillsdale: Erlbaum.

Hart, R. (2002). Introductory essay to children and young people's participation (with Gerison Lansdowne). *Special Issue of the Child Rights Information Network Newsletter, No. 16,* October, 2002. Exeter: NSPCC/Longman

Howitt, D., & Owusu-Bempah, J. (1994). *The racism of psychology: Time for change.* New York: Harvester Wheatsheaf.

Jahoda, G. (1982). *Psychology and anthropology.* London: Academic Press.

Jenks, C. (Ed.). (1982). *The sociology of childhood-essential readings.* London: Batsford.

Kağitçibaşi, C. (2007). *Family, self, and human development across cultures: Theory and applications.* Mahwah: Erlbaum.

Kishani, B.T. (2001). On the interface of philosophy and language: Some practical and theoretical considerations. *African Studies Review, 44,* 27–45.

Lanyasunya, A.R., & Lesolayia, M.S. (2001). El-barta child and family project. *Working Papers in Early Childhood Development, No. 28.* The Hague: Bernard van Leer Foundation.

Lerner, R.M. (2002). *Concepts and theories of human development* (3rd ed.). Mahwah: Erlbaum.

LeVine, R.A. (2004). Challenging expert knowledge: Findings from an African study of infant care and development. In U.P. Gielen & J. Roopnarine (Eds.), *Childhood and adolescence: Cross-cultural perspectives and applications* (pp. 149–165). Westport: Praeger.

Munday, R. (1979). 'When is a child a child?' Alternative systems of classification. *Journal of the Anthropological Society of Oxford, 10,* 161–172.

Nsamenang, A.B. (1991). *The ecology of child-care in the Bamenda Grassfields of Cameroon.* Paper presented in a Symposium on 'Ecologies of infants in different cultures,' Eleventh Biennial Meetings of the ISSBD (International Society for the Study of Behavioural Development), Minneapolis, USA.

Nsamenang, A.B. (1992a). Human development in cultural context: A third world perspective. Newbury Park: Sage.

Nsamenang, A.B. (1992b). Early childhood care and education in Cameroon. In M.E. Lamb, K.J. Sternberg, C.-P. Hwang & A.G. Broberg (Eds.), *Day care in context: Socio-cultural perspectives* (pp. 419–439). Hillsdale: Erlbaum.

Nsamenang, A.B. (2002). Adolescence in sub-Saharan Africa: An image constructed from Africa's triple inheritance. In B.B. Brown, R.W. Larson & T.S. Saraswathi (Eds.), *The world's youth: Adolescence in eight regions of the globe* (pp. 61–104). London: Cambridge University Press.

Nsamenang, A.B. (2004). *Cultures of human development and education: Challenge to growing up African.* New York: Nova.

Nsamenang, A.B. (2005). Educational development and knowledge flow: Local and global forces in human development in Africa. *Higher Education Policy, 18,* 275–288.

Nsamenang, A.B. (2006). Human ontogenesis: An indigenous African view on development and intelligence. *International Journal of Psychology, 41,* 293–297.

Nsamenang, A.B. (2008). Agency in early childhood learning and development in Cameroon. *Contemporary Issues in Early Childhood Development, 9,* 211–223.

Nsamenang, A.B. (2010). The importance of mixed age groups in Cameroon. In M. Kernan & S. Singer (Eds.), *Peer relationships in early childhood education and care* (pp. 61–73). New York: Routledge.

Nsamenang, A.B. (2011a). The culturalization of developmental trajectories: A perspective on African childhoods and adolescences. In L.A. Jensen (Ed.), *Bridging cultural and developmental approaches to psychology: New synthesis in theory, research and policy* (pp. 235–254). New York: Oxford University Press.

Nsamenang, A.B. (2011b). L'émigration clandestine des jeunes camerounais en Europe. In C. Bolzman, T.-O. Gakuba & I. Guissé (Eds.), *Migrations des jeunes d'Afrique subsaharienne: Quels defis pour l'avenir?* (pp. 139–161). Paris: L'Harmattan.

Nsamenang, A.B., & Dawes, A. (1998). Developmental psychology as political psychology in sub-Saharan Africa: The challenge of Africanisation. *Applied Psychology: An International Review, 47,* 73–87.

Nsamenang, A.B., & Lamb, M.E. (1993). The acquisition of socio-cognitive competence by Nso children in the Bamenda Grassfields of northwest Cameroon. *International Journal of Behavioral Development, 16,* 429–441.

Nsamenang, A.B., & Lamb, M.E. (1994). Socialization of Nso children in the Bamenda Grassfields of northwest Cameroon. In P.M. Greenfield & R.R. Cocking (Eds.), *Cross-cultural roots of minority child development*. Hillsdale: Erlbaum.

Nsamenang, A.B., & Lamb, M.E. (1995). The force of beliefs: How the parental values of the Nso of northwest Cameroon shape children's progress towards adult models. *Journal of Applied Developmental Psychology, 16,* 613–627.

Ochs, E. (1988). *Culture and language development*. Cambridge: Cambridge University Press.

Ogbimi, G.E., & Alao, J.A. (1998). Developing sustainable day care services in rural communities of Nigeria. *Early Child Development and Care, 145,* 47–58.

Ojiaku, M.O. (1974). Traditional African social thought and Western scholarship. *Presence Africaine, 90,* 2nd Quarterly.

Ogunaike, O.A., & Houser, Jr. R.F. (2002). Yoruba toddler's engagement inerrands and cognitive performance on the Yoruba Mental Subscale. *International Journal of Behavioral Development, 26,* 145–153.

Pence, A.R., & Hix-Small, H. (2007). Global children in the shadow of the global child. *International Journal of Educational Policy, Research and Practice, 8,* 83–100.

Pence, A.R., & Marfo, K. (2008). Early childhood development in Africa: Interrogating constraints of prevailing knowledge bases. *International Journal of Psychology, 43,* 78–87.

Pence, A.R., & Nsamenang, A.B. (2008). *A case for early child development in sub-Saharan Africa*. The Hague: BvLF.

Phinney, J.S., & Baldelomar, O.A. (2011). Identity development and multiple cultural contexts. In L.A. Jensen (Ed.), *Bridging cultural and developmental approaches to psychology: New synthesis in theory, research and policy* (pp. 161–186). New York: Oxford University Press.

Piaget, J. (1952). *The origins of intelligence in children*. New York: International Universities Press.

Prout, A., & James, A. (1990). A new paradigm for the sociology of childhood? Provenance, promise and problem. In A. James & A. Prout (Eds.), *Constructing and reconstructing childhood: Contemporary issues in the sociological study of childhood* (pp.7–34). London: The Falmer Press.

Rabain, J. (1979). *L'enfant du lignage*. Paris: Payot.

Rabain-Jamin, J. (2003). Implications of sibling caregiving for sibling relations and teaching interactions in two cultures. *Ethos, 31,* 204–231.

Reid, M. (2006). *From innocents to agents: Children and children's rights in New Zealand*. Auckland: Maxim Institute.

Richards, P. (1996). *War, youth, and resources in Sierra Leone*. Oxford: James Curry.

Rogoff, B. (2003). *The cultural nature of human development*. Oxford: Oxford University Press.

Rogoff, B., Turkanis, G.C., & Bartlett, L. (2001). *Learning together*. Oxford: Oxford University Press.

Sall, M., & Nsamenang, A.B. (2011). Ethnicity as the social foundation for education in Africa. In A.B. Nsamenang & T.M.S. Tchombe (Eds.), *Handbook of African educational theories and practices: A generative teacher education curriculum* (pp. 105–118). Yaoundé: Presses Universitaires d'Afrique.

Schildkrout, E. (1978). Age and gender in Hausa society: Socio-economic roles of children in urban Kano. In J.S. LaFontaine (Ed.), *Age and sex as principles of social differentiation* (pp. 109–136). London: Academic Press.

Serpell, R. (1993). *The significance of schooling: Life-journeys into an African society*. Cambridge: Cambridge University Press.

Serpell, R. (1994). An African social ontogeny: Review of A. Bame Nsamenang (1992): Human development in cultural context. *Cross-Cultural Psychology Bulletin, 28,* 17–21.

Serpell, R. (2008). Participatory appropriation and the cultivation of nurturance: A case study of African primary school health science curriculum development. In P.R. Dasen & A. Akkari (Eds.), *Educational theories and practices from the 'majority world'* (pp. 71–97). New Delhi: Sage.

Skovdal, M., Ogutu, V., Aoro, C., & Campbell, C. (2009). Young carers as social actors: coping strategies of children caring for ailing or ageing guardians in Western Kenya. *Social Science & Medicine, 69,* 587–595.

Slavin, R.E. (1987). Developmental and motivational perspectives on cooperative learning: Reconciliation. *Child Development, 58,* 1161–1167.

Smith, P.B., Bond, M.H., & Kağıtçıbaşi, C. (2006). *Understanding social psychology across cultures*. London: Sage.

Solberg, A. (1995). Negotiating childhood: Changing constructions of age for Norwegian children. In A. James & A. Prout (Eds.), *Constructing and reconstructing childhood*. London: Falmer Press.

Steinberg, S.R., & Kincheloe, J.L. (2004). *Kinderculture: The corporate construction of childhood*. Boulder, CO: Westview Press Inc.

UNESCO (1999). UNESCO World Conference on Science Declaration on Science and the Use of Scientific Knowledge. Retrieved on 4/24/2003, from http://www.unesco.org.

UNICEF (2003). *Convention on the Rights of the Child*. Available from www.unicef.org/crc/crc.htm.

Vygotsky, L. (1978). *Mind in society: The development of higher psychological processes*. Cambridge: Cambridge University Press.

Ware, H. (1983). Male and female life cycles. In C. Oppong (Ed.), *Male and female in West Africa* (pp. 6–31). London: Allen & Unwin.

Weisner, T.S. (1987). Socialization for parenthood in sibling caretaking societies. In J.B. Lancaster, J. Altman, A.S. Rossi & L.R. Sherrod (Eds.), *Parenting across the lifespan: Biosocial dimensions* (pp. 237–270). Hawthorne: Aldine de Gruyter.

Woodhead, M. (2008). Identity at birth – and identity in development. In L. Brooker & M. Woodhead (Eds.), *Developing positive identities: Early Childhood in Focus 3 (Diversity and Young Children)* (p. 4). Walton Hall, Milton Keynes: The Open University.

Zelizer, V. (1985). *Pricing the priceless child: The changing social value of children*. New York: Basic Books.

Zimba, R.F. (2002). Indigenous conceptions of childhood development and social realities in southern Africa. In H. Keller, Y.P. Poortinga & A. Scholmerish (Eds.), *Between cultures and biology: Perspectives on ontogenetic development* (pp. 89–115). Cambridge: Cambridge University Press.

Zornado, J.L. (2001). *Inventing the child: Culture, ideology, and the story of childhood*. New York: Garland.

A. Bame Nsamenang
Director, Human Development Resource Centre (HDRC)
P.O. Box 270
Bamenda, North West Region (Cameroon)
Tel. +237 7725 4133, E-Mail bame@thehdrc.org

A. Bame Nsamenang (PhD 1984, University of Ibadan, Nigeria) is associate professor of psychology and learning science at the University of Bamenda, Cameroon, and founding director of Human Development Resource Centre, a research and service facility for future generations – children and youth. His research seeks to understand and enhance their development in context. He networks for African voices into developmental science discourses and literature and leads an initiative that produces Africa-centric literature and tools for early childhood development and teacher education (see www.thehdrc.org).

Commentary

Slaughter-Defoe DT (ed): Racial Stereotyping and Child Development.
Contrib Hum Dev. Basel, Karger, 2012, vol 25, pp 105–108

On Researching the Agency of Youth: Moving Beyond Traditional Theorizing

Commentary on Nsamenang

Celine I. Thompson

University of Pennsylvania, Graduate School of Education, Applied Psychology and Human Development Division,
Philadelphia, Pa., USA

As with just about any field dedicated to scientific research, developmental science benefits from theories and ideas that question any hegemonic monocultural views that tend to dominate how we conceptualize human behavior. Professor Nsamenang provides this audience with ideas and evidence that make it clear that the traditional ways of understanding youth development inadequately function as the only tool in our research repertoire. As he explains why our conceptions of youth development must reach beyond traditional Eurocentric and Western views, it becomes evident that research in human development needs more than just additional monocultural views of what healthy human development should look like. We need theories and research paradigms that no longer find it sufficient to question the need to consider cultural variation, but instead incorporate human phenomenology into theoretical frameworks. It is because of this need that this reader begs the question: Are we not supported with enough evidence to topple the prominent tower of Western views and replace them with concepts that inherently acknowledge, accept and value cultural variation? Nsamenang provides the rhetorical response to this query as he describes African youth agency in their development, particularly in the family realm. Beyond any specific view of healthy youth developmental outcomes and processes, he makes it apparent that any ultimate or dominant perspective that governs developmental science research should be guided by the cultural setting of the subject of inquiry.

Learning in Nonacademic Contexts from Peers and Family Members

Demonstration of the need for embracing non-traditional theoretical perspectives is witnessed in Nsamenang's description of the importance of learning in the peer and family realm compared to the exclusive focus on academic enhancement. He goes on to describe how children's agency invokes 'dependence, interdependence, vulnerability, need, and development' [p. 94], something that traditional schooling may not afford them. These qualities may help African youth 'navigate the harsh realities of their circumstances' to achieve successfully according to the needs and expectations of their own communities and societies. Nsamenang accomplishes two specific tasks in his description of child agency in Africentric human development. First, he establishes the child as an active participant in his or her development. Children are not described as static beings, maturing in block-level stages with specific tasks assigned to and expected from them at each level. The gradual development that Nsamenang illustrates provides flexibility in how children can learn and become proficient within their families and communities, not just academically. Additionally, his view inherently acknowledges, accepts, and values the role of peer interaction in development! This mere and subtle inclusion of the role of peer cultures in youth development establishes the need for extending our perceptions beyond exclusive adult-child interactions in accomplishing developmental tasks.

Second, by not focusing exclusively on academic tasks, Nsamenang highlights the importance of 'the social, emotional, practical, cognitive, relational values and other norms ingrained in the activity settings of the home, society, and peer cultures' [p. 95]. The value of family and peer expectations for behavior and proficiency in home, society, and peer contexts is immeasurable in terms of significance in agentive child development as described by Nsamenang. He seems to emphasize the notion that healthy youth development is less dependent upon accomplishing proficiency in specific academic tasks, and more focused on a comprehensive cultural expectation of youth development. This view is more dynamic and can be tailored to any cultural group, without need for subscribed allegiance to any one philosophy, traditional or otherwise. Nsamenang outlines clearly the differences in Western and Africentric views of outcomes and expectations for youth development, and this suggests that the research community can comfortably adopt views of human development that contrast with and diverge from the traditional. To take things a step further, our engagement in human development research, particularly youth development research, could benefit from approaches that seek to develop theories and perspectives derived from focusing on specific youth experiences. One important way in which we can accomplish this goal in developmental science research is by shifting our focus on the cultural expectations youth are perceived as required to perform and acknowledging the role of multiple contexts in socializing these expectations upon our youth. To begin this worthy task, we have to allow indigenous cultural settings the right to determine what healthy development looks like.

Childhood Adultification

Professor Nsamenang provides a useful example for brief discussion of cultural interpretation of what is 'healthy' youth development. His description and explanation of youth participation in family duties is one that frames those behaviors as learning activities. However, depending upon how one views child involvement in family duties, these 'caring roles and socially and economically productive activities' [p. 94] could easily be viewed as softer-hued childhood adultification. Burton [2007] associates childhood adultification with economic disadvantage; childhood adultification is viewed more as a consequence of some deficit caused by adversity. The child takes on a role that the parent would primarily assume that of caregiver and sometimes, provider as well. It is generally presumed to be an unhealthy way for youth to behave, causing them stress and negative outcomes [Allison et al., 1999; Burton, 2007; Jones & Trickett, 2005]. Nsamenang's emphasis on the agency of youth to engage in what is described as 'family duties', not adult-exclusive activity, allows conceptualization of how beneficial these activities are for youth development, instead of focusing primarily on how such behavior is harmful and indicative of dysfunctional development. By asserting that the family duties children perform strengthen their own skills as maturing citizens, attention is focused on growth and nurturance, instead of deficit and stunted experience. Childhood adultification is conceived as a phenomenon born out of need, and little research has focused on its benefits for youth [Jones & Trickett, 2005]. It is as if a taint covers the utility of youth within their families when it is perceived as adultification; however, Nsamenang presents the help that African youth provide in the same context as a normal, healthy and *expected* experience. The social and emotional benefits of participating in family and household duties for youth are underexplored. Nsamenang presents a sanguine perspective of youth agentive engagement in human development that adds to how we can perceive and study the effects of youth participation within the family realm.

Understanding the Emergence of Self-Identity in Nontraditional Contexts

The task of adopting divergent and healthy perspectives of African youth development is accomplished by Nsamenang; however, its extension to global views of youth identity development could benefit from clarification on how it is influenced by participation in family and community realms. Nsamenang situates the process of self-identity as one that is neither exclusively individual nor connected. Social context makes this process more complex than assuming that any individual could view themselves as completely autonomous or completely interconnected. If youth are 'systematically socialized and educated, if not indoctrinated, into being interconnected to or detached from social others,' [p. 96] then the external social world ascribes norms that shape the process of self-identity. Simply stated, it is the child's social context that primarily decides what is 'meaningful'

about their sense of identity. Nsamenang mentions the significance of group affiliation helping 'people define themselves in the eyes of others and themselves' [p. 97]. Group membership has an influential role in how any youth develops lenses to view themselves as individuals.

The next step to understanding how one engages in the process of self-identity is to consider the intersectional impact of membership in multiple groups. Immigrant status, racial group, gender, sexual orientation, disability, economic status, tribal affiliation, etc., shape the ways in which youth view themselves in the world around them. Additionally, societal, familial, tribal, racial and ethnic traditions and norms provide expectations for individuals who belong to any and all of these groups. One approach that future developmental research can adopt to gain a more complete picture of healthy youth development is to acknowledge the existence and influence of these intersecting identities. Theoretical frameworks that rely on social context as the basis for approaching developmental science research can avoid the pitfalls of the dominant, yet limited monocultural perspectives of healthy human development. It increases the observation of agency of youth in their own development, credits socializing parties other than parents for their role in shaping identity formation, and holds researchers accountable for how they conceptualize 'healthy development', just to consider a few possibilities. Rhetorically speaking, do we finally have enough reason and evidence to move beyond the task of disproving Eurocentric theoretical dominance and instead invest energy in explaining culturally-nuanced healthy human development?

References

Allison, K.W., Burton, L., Marshall, S., Perez-Febles, A., Yarrington, J., Kirsh, L.B., & Merriwether-DeVries, C. (1999). Life experiences among urban adolescents: Examining the role of context. *Child Development, 70,* 1017–1029.

Burton, L. (2007). Childhood adultification in economically disadvantaged families: A conceptual model. *Family Relations: An Interdisciplinary Journal of Applied Family Studies, 56,* 329–345.

Jones, C.J., & Trickett, E.J. (2005). Immigrant adolescents behaving as culture brokers: A study of families from the former Soviet Union. *The Journal of Social Psychology, 145,* 405–427.

Celine I. Thompson
University of Pennsylvania, Graduate School of Education, Applied Psychology and Human Development Division
3700 Walnut Street
Philadelphia, PA 19104 (USA)
E-Mail celineithompson@gmail.com

Ms. Celine I. Thompson (PhD Candidate, Applied Psychology and Human Development, University of Pennsylvania) received her Bachelor of Arts degree in Psychology, minor in Afro-American Studies, and a Master of Science in Education degree from the University of Pennsylvania. As a current doctoral candidate in the Interdisciplinary Studies in Human Development program at the Graduate School of Education at the University of Pennsylvania, she is currently working on her dissertation focusing on identity development from a 'racially-gendered' intersectional perspective in Black female adolescents. Her other research interests include understanding student perspectives of social justice issues in the classroom.

Commentary

Slaughter-Defoe DT (ed): Racial Stereotyping and Child Development.
Contrib Hum Dev. Basel, Karger, 2012, vol 25, pp 109–112

Advancing an African Research Agenda for Child Development

Commentary on Nsamenang

Katie Maeve Murphy

University of Pennsylvania, Philadelphia, Pa., USA

Contributions from European and North American research have described child development as change spurred by interactional processes between a child and her environment occurring within a complex ecosystem that encapsulates families, communities and the broader social and political contexts [Bronfenbrenner, 1986]. With little variation, the epicenter of this ecosystem is the individual child, engulfed by the child's most powerful sphere of influence – the parents, and more specifically the mother. As asserted by Professor Nsamenang, this 'Western' conception ignores the important role of siblings, extended families, and multi-age, multi-sex peer groups thereby undermining the powerful role of children's agency in African societies. Highlighting the need for research grounded in the African context conducted by African scholars, Nsamenang points to the collective processes of learning and socialization occurring within polycultural groups of children, as opposed to the egocentric emphasis on individual development touted by Western theories [pp. 90, 100].

While recognizing the undeniable need for Africentric research to further explore and analyze the processes of learning and socialization within multi-age, multi-sex groups of children and siblings, several critical issues warrant a focused attention. These include within-country and within-community variations in the structures of multi-age, multi-sex group learning and socialization and the patterns of sibling-care that may impact schooling, especially for girls. At the same time, the focus on the particular African context need not ignore insights offered by research from other regions of the world, as the phenomenon of multi-age groups of children engaged in caretaking, playing, working and learning has been observed throughout the world, particularly in agrarian societies (e.g., Whiting's studies of sibling care giving in Guatemala India, Japan, Kenya, Mexico, Peru, the Philippines, and the United States, described in Whiting and Edwards [1988], or Maynard's study of cultural teaching through sibling interactions in Zinacantec Mayan children in Maynard [2002]). Although Professor Nsamenang demonstrates an awareness of such studies, his discussion of African children stresses a divergence from existing research, thereby failing to point out some of the important similarities that may be found in various societies throughout the world.

Exploring Variations

As a continent that contains hundreds of ethno-linguistic groups spread across a broad diversity of agro-ecological zones and socioeconomic conditions, Africa resists generalizations. Thus, the assertion of a distinctly Pan-African conception of child development requires a close analysis of the variations in the dynamic systems of caretaking, socialization and learning in order to assert a unique, African experience. In several instances, Nsamenang acknowledges Africa's rich and complex diversity as he underscores the role of ethnicity and culture in the formation of identity [pp. 96–97] and as he articulates the need for an increased understanding of a variety of childhood experiences across cultures rather than employing a universal application of Western theories [p. 100]. Nonetheless, he persistently maintains an interest in describing a macro-level view of the characteristics and developmental processes of the 'African' child [e.g. pp. 90, 95, 96, 97, 101]. In this sense, there does not seem to be a move toward understanding the variety of childhood experiences, but instead a substitution of Western theory with a universal 'African' theory.

The primary sources of Professor Nsamenang's findings are based on cohort studies of Nso families in Cameroon, followed by subsequent observational studies of Nso infants in rural and urban settings [pp. 91, 99] as well as highlights from research conducted primarily in Kenya and Nigeria. While similarities across Africa may certainly exist, important variations would likely be observed across a diversity of ethnic groups in rural compared to urban settings, in wealthy compared to poorer households and even within small, seemingly homogenous communities. Traditional community and familial power structures, relative differences in wealth, and exposures to Western values emphasizing dyadic relationships and individual development may influence caretaking practices and the strength and configuration of children's relationships with peers and family

members. An exploration of these variations may provide support for the Pan-African model, but it may also reveal significant correlates of sibling and multi-age group care, such as wealth, fertility rates, dependence on small-scale agriculture or subsistence farming and other community demographics. If such correlates exist, the conceptualization of the Pan-African model of child development may warrant revision in order to provide a more inclusive and complete picture of the contemporary African child's experience across a broad range of settings.

Children's Agency in Sibling-Care and the Gender Factor

Nsamenang describes children as active agents of their own learning, highlighting the need to further understand these 'nonacademic pathways' of social, cultural and cognitive growth and the 'agentive strategies with which African children navigate the harsh realities of their circumstances to survive and make progress on their own devices' [p. 93]. He aptly points out the failure of formal education systems based on colonial legacies in recognizing the skills and values inherent in traditional societies [p. 93]. At the same time, Nsamenang suggests that family-based education and multi-age, multi-sex peer group interactions serve as a complement to formal schooling [p. 93].

This important point requires further investigation to ensure that opportunities for schooling are not compromised by participation in sibling care and peer group activities, especially for girls who may often carry a disproportionate share of caretaking responsibilities. For example, studies from Ghana and India suggest that sibling care has a negative effect on girls' schooling. In Ghana, Lloyd and Gage-Brandon [1992] investigated the relationship between family size and educational attainment based on the 1987 Ghana Living Measurements Standards Survey. For a girl enrolled in school, the study found that each increase in the number of younger siblings resulted in a significant increase in the likelihood that the girl would drop out of school. For boys enrolled in school, there was no significant association between education and number of younger siblings, indicating that girls may carry the majority of the burden of sibling care in Ghana, and that sibling care often *replaces* rather than *complements* formal schooling. Similarly in India, research has found that approximately 54% of girls do not attend school due to family obligations to provide sibling care, while only 8% of boys reportedly do not attend school due to sibling care [PROBE Team, 1999].

It can be argued that traditional learning through peers and family members provides an opportunity to develop skills that cannot be learned in school, and these non-school experiences may be critical for developing creativity, ingenuity and technological skills necessary to thrive within a particular community. Nonetheless, a substantial body of research connects educational attainment in Africa with future increases in health and income [e.g., Psacharopoulos, 2004], and therefore it is important to understand the developmental outcomes for the older children who assume leadership roles in multi-age, multi-sex peer groups, and the impact this has on their educational outcomes. Thus, without denying the value of non-school learning, further investigations are required to ensure that girls' participation in schooling is not threatened by their important role in sibling care, so that they too may have the opportunity to pursue education as a means for achieving improved economic and social outcomes [Slaughter-Defoe, Addae & Bell, 2002].

Conclusion

Drawing from research deeply contextualized in childhood experiences in distinct African societies, Professor Nsamenang presents new insights into the inadequacy of traditional Western conceptualizations of child development in describing the complex processes of collaborative group learning, family-based education and multi-age, multi-sex interactions. Pointing to the dearth of rigorous, Africentric research on the subject, the paper presents a powerful call to action for child development research within the African context. As posited in this response, such research should include a careful analysis of the variations in traditional systems for learning and socialization across the multitude of distinct contexts within Africa, and should consider the impact that participation in peer group learning has on developmental outcomes for the children (especially girls) who are charged with the responsibility of assuming a leadership role in care giving activities. Advancing this research agenda would provide valuable and much needed contributions to the field of Child Development in Africa, and could potentially provide a contextualized framework for understanding and assessing holistic child development in African societies.

References

Bronfenbrenner, U. (1986). Ecology of the family as a context for human development: Research perspectives. *Developmental Psychology, 22,* 723–742.

Lloyd, C.B., & Gage-Brandon, A.J. (1992). *Does subsize matter? The implications of family size for children's education in Ghana, Working Paper No. 45.* New York: The Population Council.

Maynard, A.E. (2002). Cultural teaching: The development of teaching skills in Maya sibling interactions. *Child Development, 73,* 969–982.

PROBE Team, The (1999). *PROBE: Public Report on Basic Education in India.* New Delhi: Oxford University Press.

Psacharopoulos, G. (2004). Returns to investment in education: a further update. *Education Economics, 12(2)*, 111–134.

Slaughter-Defoe, D., Addae, W.A., & Bell, C. (2002). Toward the future schooling of girls: Global status, issues, and prospects. *Human Development, 45,* 34–53.

Whiting, B.B., & Edwards, C.P. (1988). *Children of different worlds: The formation of social behavior*. Cambridge: Harvard University Press.

Katie Maeve Murphy
University of Pennsylvania
3700 Walnut Street
Philadelphia, PA 19104–6216 (USA)
E-Mail kmaeve@gmail.com

Ms. Katie Maeve Murphy (M.Ed., International Education Policy, Harvard University) is a joint PhD and MPH student in Interdisciplinary Studies in Human Development at the University of Pennsylvania, focusing on holistic interventions to improve developmental, educational, and health outcomes for children in low-income and impoverished settings. Katie was a health, sanitation, and education volunteer with the Peace Corps in El Salvador, where she lived in a rural community for 2 years working in education, health and income generation. Recently, Katie conducted research on early childhood development in India and Thailand, and she has worked and traveled extensively throughout Latin America, South Asia and Southeast Asia, and Africa, visiting over 10 countries in sub-Saharan Africa while working on education initiatives at the Earth Institute. Katie also lived in Northeastern Chad and worked with Darfurian and Chadian children, youth, parents, and teachers as the Education Manager for the International Rescue Committee (10/2005–4/2006).

Slaughter-Defoe DT (ed): Racial Stereotyping and Child Development.
Contrib Hum Dev. Basel, Karger, 2012, vol 25, pp 113–115

Epilogue

Diana T. Slaughter-Defoe

University of Pennsylvania, Philadelphia, Pa., USA

This Epilogue highlights some important points made in this volume that I, as editor, believe readers may overlook or take for granted when in fact some attention to them will likely reinvigorate and energize studies of culture, race, and racial attitudes and stereotyping. Including the stimulating chapter by Professor Nsamenang in this volume, for example, reminds us that to date studies of racial attitudes and stereotyping have primarily focused on geographical contexts in which Blacks are racial and ethnic minorities. However, racial stereotyping has and can occur within majority-Black contexts as Professor Nsamenang so ably argues. While he would definitely agree with Professor Burton [Burton, 2007] that childhood adultification does exist in economically disadvantaged contexts, he would definitely *not* agree with Burton's analysis that its presence has only or even primarily negative consequences. Commentators Thompson, and Murphy, both pursuing doctoral studies at the University of Pennsylvania, point to how cultures and genders within cultures may be differentially affected by race-related stereotyped roles.

Chappell reported that a new book by Tina Wells, *Chasing youth culture and getting it right*, advocates marketing to teen 'mind-sets' instead of teen demographics such as youth, aged 13–19: 'Wells divided (US) youth into four groups or 'tribes': independents, preppies, techies and alternatives. Figuring out how to market to these groups is the challenge. . .' [Chappell, 2011, p. 68]. This analysis is consistent with the research findings of Adams and Stevenson that emphasize measurement of the interaction between individual social cognitive processes and perceptible, externalized racial attitudes and stereotypes. Two commentators on the chapter by Adams and Stevenson, Pieotrowski and Jones, stress the conceptual and methodological complexities involved in conducting important future basic and applied research in this area. Cultures, already diverse, change and thus do the mindsets of their youth. Importantly, thanks to the Internet (Matwyshyn) social media are more diverse today than historically ever before, and the actual and potential worldwide reach is considerably expanded (note the reach of 'You-Tube' for example.). As Johnson observed in the Commentary to the chapter by Bogan and Slaughter-Defoe, we can expect data gathering on the topic of racial attitudes and stereotyping for some time to come. I strongly agree with the Commentary of Bigler and Wright: It is too early in the research to forecast remedies – we have much to learn, and I think the area can be advanced by international and intercultural collaborative research.

Consider, for example, the data obtained between Black and White US youth as reported in Bogan and Slaughter-Defoe's chapter. In fact, we know from both chapters by Slaughter-Defoe and co-workers that recent research has identified potential linkages between social psychological variables known to impact Black students' school achievement (e.g., 'stereotype threat', a concept advanced by Claude Steele [2004]) and culturally based racial stereotypes. Bogan and colleagues report that linkages are absent within samples of White youth, but pronounced among Black youth. English-Clarke and colleagues report that adolescent Black youth could appraise their own mathematical capabilities in accordance with perceptions of early stories, favorable or unfavorably rendered (see the important Commentary by Beale Spencer) by extended family members, their friends and teachers. These are new but still exploratory findings that greatly expand upon earlier, simplistic notions of linkages only between Black children's racial attitudes and their self-esteem [Slaughter-Defoe, Johnson & Spencer, 2009]. Further, as noted in the Commentaries of McGee and Miller and Bracey, fine-tuning of study methods is definitely indicated, including through creative, observation-based future studies.

Contemporary anthropologically oriented scholars of race undoubtedly owe a huge debt to Franz Boas. According to Baker [1998], 'In anthropology, the leading spokesperson against Social Darwinism and for liberal reform was Franz Boas, in sociology, W.E.B. Du Bois. During the first decade of the 20th century, Boas. . . effectively directed the anthropology of race away from theories of evolution and guided it to a consensus that African Americans, Native Americans, and other people of color were not racially inferior and possessed unique and historically specific cultures. . . particular to geographic areas, local histories, and traditions. . . cultures were relative. . .' [Baker, pp. 99–100].

Nonetheless, decades of social and scientific struggle still have not achieved complete consensus on this principle. I believe the emergence of significant, though small, cadres of racial and ethnic minority scientists in the last half of the 20th century contributed heavily to the propagation of the liberal ideas of scholars like Boas and W.E. B. Du Bois [Holliday, 2009; Holliday & Holmes, 2003; Slaughter-Defoe, Garrett & Harrison, 2006; Spencer, Brookins & Allen, 1985] in the human development field, generally, and child development in particular. Ultimately, scientists and scholars of all races instigated and contributed to this important paradigm shift: We now understand that stereotyping of children of African descent, whether they are of minority or majority status sociocultural context occurs partly because (a) cultural traditions of non-Western origins are not appreciated, and (b) child individuation within the parental and family home environment does not encapsulate all forms of identity development. In large numbers of contemporary communities and societies, identity is co-constructed with extended family members *and* with peers and potent media sources.

References

Baker, L.D. (1998). *From savage to Negro: Anthropology and the construction of race, 1896–1954.* Berkeley: University of California Press.

Burton, L. (2007). Childhood adultification in economically disadvantaged families: A conceptual model. *Family Relations, 56,* 329–345.

Chappel, K. (2011). Tapping into the youth market. *Ebony Magazine, Vol. LXVI,* 67–68.

Holliday, B.G. (2009). The history and visions of African American psychology: Multiple pathways to place, space, and authority. *Cultural diversity and ethnic minority psychology, 15,* 317–337.

Holliday, B.G., & Holmes, A.L. (2003). A tale of challenge and change: A history and chronology of ethnic minorities in the United States. In G. Bernal, J. Trimble, A.K. Burlew & F. Leong (Eds.), *Handbook of racial and ethnic minority psychology* (pp. 15–59). Thousand Oaks, CA: Sage Publications, Inc.

Slaughter-Defoe, D.T., Garrett, A.M., & Harrison-Hale, A.O. (2006). Our children too: A history of the Black Caucus of the Society for Research in Child Development, 1973–1997. S.L. Graham, Series Guest Ed., *Monographs of the Society for Research in Child Development*, Serial No. 283, 71.

Slaughter-Defoe, D.T., Johnson, D.J., & Spencer, M.B. (2009). Race and children's development. In R.A. Shweder, T.R. Bidell, A.C. Dailey, S.D. Dixon, P.J. Miller & J. Modell (Eds.), *The child: An encyclopedic companion* (pp. 801–806). Chicago: University of Chicago Press.

Spencer, M.B., Brookins, G.K., & Allen, W.R. (1985). *Beginnings: The social and affective development of Black children*. Hillsdale: Lawrence Erlbaum Associates.

Steele, C. (2004). A threat in the air: How stereotypes shape intellectual identity and performance. In J.A. Banks & C.A.M. Banks (Eds.), *Handbook of research on multicultural education* (2nd ed., pp. 682–699). San Francisco: Jossey-Bass.

Prof. Diana T. Slaughter-Defoe
Graduate School of Education
The University of Pennsylvania
3700 Walnut Street
Philadelphia, PA 19104–6216 (USA)
Tel. +1 215 582 7036
E-Mail dianasd@gse.upenn.edu

Dr. Diana T. Slaughter-Defoe (PhD 1968, University of Chicago) received her doctorate from the Committee on Human Development in developmental and clinical psychology, and is presently the Constance E. Clayton Professor Emerita in the Graduate School of Education at the University of Pennsylvania. Her research interests have included culture, primary education, and home-school relations facilitating in-school academic achievement. Since retirement, she has also edited: *Black Educational Choice: Assessing the Private and Public Alternatives to K-12 Public Schools* [Praeger, 2011] with colleagues, and *Messages for Educational Leadership: The Constance E. Clayton Lectures, 1998–2007* [Peter Lang Publishers, 2012]. She is presently writing a memoir about her career that spanned 40-plus years in academia and higher education.

Author Index

Subject Index